T0085888

Breast Cancer and Iodine

By
David M. Derry, M.D., Ph.D.

The author welcomes your comments at dderry@shaw.ca

National Library of Canada Cataloguing in Publication Data

Derry, David M. (David Michael), 1937-
  Breast cancer and iodine

ISBN 1-55212-884-9

1. Breast--Cancer--Popular works. I. Title.
RC280.B8D47 2001   616.99'449   C2001-911174-6

TRAFFORD

This book was published *on-demand* in cooperation with Trafford Publishing.
On-demand publishing is a unique process and service of making a book available for retail sale to the public taking advantage of on-demand manufacturing and Internet marketing.
On-demand publishing includes promotions, retail sales, manufacturing, order fulfilment, accounting and collecting royalties on behalf of the author.

Suite 6E, 2333 Government St., Victoria, B.C. V8T 4P4, CANADA
Phone   250-383-6864   Toll-free   1-888-232-4444 (Canada & US)
Fax   250-383-6804   E-mail   sales@trafford.com
Web site   www.trafford.com   TRAFFORD PUBLISHING IS A DIVISION OF TRAFFORD HOLDINGS LTD.
Trafford Catalogue #01-0286   www.trafford.com/robots/01-0286.html

10   9   8   7   6   5

Acknowledgements:

My wife Pat, my soul mate, is in every sense of the word the
reason for this book.

Two others have been important sounding boards to the
development of the concepts;

Marjorie McKinnon and Frankie Staples.
Kudos for all your efforts.

Author's note

This book is a theoretical discussion, and has also been produced to provide information and discussions of different ideas about approaches to breast cancer. Some examples of anecdotal results have been discussed but are not meant to imply that the results were more than that. The theories put forward here are testable in the time-honoured manner of proper studies with adequate numbers of people to make the statistics significant.

We know that all significant new ideas or approaches to difficult problems have to start somewhere with one patient. This may be planned or accidental. From there perhaps a tentative theory may be formed and the concept re-tried on another patient. Over time and with a knowledge of the longer-term anecdotal results, we can get a feel for the validity of new ideas. General Practitioners are in the best position medically to examine the results of all treatments. By the nature of their relation to the patient they can watch not only the effect of the treatment, but also all of the other factors which may influence the outcome.

Not only is this book incomplete, but some aspects of the theories are still evolving on the basis of further experience. At some point during a process of investigation, however, one has to sit down and say something about where we are. It doesn't mean that we have the answers, but that this is what is thought at this point. This book is therefore really the prologue to a larger edition. Time has been the main factor preventing me from making this book as complete and detailed as I would like. The purpose of it is to stir up discussion of the difficult and complex problem of breast cancer and cancer in general.

Because there is a distinct lack of comprehensive theories about the mechanisms of cancer, no real effort has been made in this book to compare competing theories. In fact, in most instances of discussion by world authorities, comparison of theories has been discouraged because of cancer's complexity, multiplicity of causes, and variability of clinical and microscopic outcomes.

I do not feel we should be discouraged from trying. Theories are what allow scientists to explore nature with eyes and brains that are more focussed. Even if a theory is shown to be wrong and stimulates thought, the new research vigor can lead to a more correct theory. Competing theories may lead to more rapid advancement of research programs toward the real goal of conquering cancer. Thus, the information presented herein is in no way intended as a substitute for proper medical advice from the reader's physician. If this book serves to stimulate discussion, it will have served its purpose at his time.

Table of contents

Introduction

This book is about the cause, prevention and treatment of breast cancer. Over the last century enough data and observations have become available to allow the collection of this material into a coherent, understandable and testable thesis of how breast cancer starts and how it progresses. This monograph therefore is devoted to the exploration of a new outlook towards breast cancer with passing mention of related cancers and diseases. When discussing cancer we are talking about a systemic process, which allows the development of a predictable sequence of biological changes leading to cancer. This presentation is not meant to be exhaustive, and I hope to complete a more comprehensive treatment of this thesis in the future. Purposely, I have addressed this book to women with breast cancer. Since reading some of the stories of personal experiences with breast cancer, I am full of admiration for the knowledge and enthusiasm with which they pursue this disease and the research connected with it.

Part of the present participation by women is related to the activism which accompanied the AIDS disease outbreak. For the first time women saw that they too had a place in the decision making and began to influence research funding towards projects they instinctively knew needed exploring. This is admirable, because academic research cannot always see obvious holes in the research fields, and they may not be able or interested in filling in those holes. It is hard to get away from breast cancer statistics, such as, unchanged mortality rates since the records were kept in the 1920s. Also discouraging, are the newly designed detection and screening methods, which seem to fail in changing disease outcomes. It is even disappointing that old fashion self examination appears not to help with survival. These discouraging results and statistics may only be the result of a lack of a coherent understandable theory of the cause of breast cancer so that a clean new approach to the disease can be started. Slowly different exploratory approaches to breast cancer are emerging from the periphery of the present established cancer understanding, but none yet show a clear opening to crack the mystery of this disease. It is hoped that this little presentation will give food for thought and maybe lead to some further advances.

The monograph is divided into four parts:

1. Iodine and its evolution and role in the cell
2. Iodine and thyroid hormone and its relations to the patient's constitution
3. Cancer in general as a process.
4. Breast cancer fibrocystic disease, its prevention and arrest.

The first part is information on iodine and its relation to the body and thyroid gland. Iodine appears to be the least understood important element making up the body fluids and cells of humans. Iodine has been neglected, as huge amounts of research funds have not uncovered any other function of iodine than that it makes thyroid hormone and it serves as an excellent antiseptic, which we have known for more than a hundred years. In spite of all the research we do not know what biochemical processes it participates in or what part it plays in the overall metabolism of the body other than its role in the formation of thyroid hormone.

I propose primarily that iodine is the trigger mechanism for apoptosis (the natural death of cells) and the main surveillance mechanism for abnormal cells in the body. Iodine triggers the death of cells which are abnormal or which have normal programmed death as part of their life cycle. This is part of a general thesis that iodine and thyroid hormone act as a team to provide a constant surveillance against abnormal cell development, chemicals that are carcinogenic and the spread of cancer cells within the body. Iodine appears to have several more roles in the body. Iodine protects against abnormal growth of bacteria in the stomach (helicobacter pylori is the most clinically significant). Iodine can coat incoming allergic proteins to make them non-allergic, which likely also applies to the internal equivalent called autoimmune disease. Iodine binds softly to the double and triple bond of lipids to protect these bonds while they are being transported to synaptic sites in the brain and blood vessels of the body. As well iodine in the stomach deactivates all biological and most chemical poisons. All of these new proposed testable functions of iodine are discussed. There is a discussion of the possible role of iodine in evolution in relation to development of multi-cellularity and maturation of vertebrates The general thesis of this book is that there is a specific dose of iodine intake above which it prevents several disease processes including those related to fibrocystic disease and breast cancer

The second part is related to the thyroid hormones and the thyroid gland. In both of these first two sections some suggestions as to the evolutionary source of iodine and thyroid hormone are outlined. From here we can understand that tissue levels of thyroid hormone are just as important if not more important than circulating blood levels. It is proposed that thyroid hormone has controlled the genome (Nuclear DNA sequences etc) since the beginning. Because of this, control of intracellular low levels of thyroid hormone would tend to let genes, which can cause disease, to escape and express themselves. Therefore thyroid hormone's main purpose, aside from keeping the genome stable, is to run each of the cells in relation to each other and also to permissively allow other hormones to act.

Thyroid hormone came well before any of the other hormones and has taken up the position of the most important hormone. Since iodine came before thyroid hormone, then iodine is more important than the hormone. Some of the clinical aspects of thyroid hormone treatment are discussed in relation to disturbances in the receptor mechanisms and its relation to thyroid hormone resistance.

The third part deals largely with the findings of the intensive cancer investigations of the last 60 years or more. The late Dr. David Clarke Jr. wrote some detailed thoughts on the biological development of the cancer process. Now, along with findings by Dr. Sampson of the Mayo clinic in the 1970s, it becomes evident that perhaps cancer is a biphasic process (two phases). More clearly stated, cancer has two phases. The first is controlled by iodine up to the phenomena called "carcinoma in situ" or "occult cancer" and thyroid hormone seems to control the second phase, namely the spread of cancer within connective tissues.

The forth and last part concerns the application of the first three parts to breast cancer. Much of the material in this part of the book seems to fall into place if the postulates put forward are legitimately representing what is happening in this disease. With these concepts we can relate the risk factors and epidemiological studies on breast cancer to prevention and treatment.

On a personal note I want to explain briefly my route to this book. Having become highly trained and qualified to do basic research, domestic re-arrangements made pursuit of this career a financial impossibility. Hence I had a complete career change in 1972, from academic halls to the front lines of general practice. It was my over-riding philosophy when I entered general practice that I would learn and practice to listen to the patient. Sir William Osler said it clearly but Syndenham said it first, that if you listen to the patient they will tell you the diagnosis and if you listen even more closely they will tell you the correct treatment. I have tried to hone my skills in this one area of medicine and found it to be a gold mine of interesting new concepts.

Iodine

Iodine is the only chemical element having two meteoric rises, 100 years apart, in popularity in the general population and the medical establishment. At the same time, iodine is one of the few elements that has fallen to such scientific obscurity in spite of its importance to vertebrates, especially humans

Yet, there are comprehensive texts on iodine metabolism, thyroid gland and hormones. Also, there are extensive studies on iodine deficiency and well known textbooks of endocrinology. Every cell and every fluid of the vertebrate body contains iodine, so it is surprising to learn few biological textbooks have iodine in their index.

Iodine's discovery

Iodine's rise to fame as one of the greatest panaceas of all time occurred not many years after it was discovered in about 1811. After all, iodine was the first single element curing a particular disease, namely goiter (swelling of the thyroid gland). Since iodine is a non—metallic essential element that never appears in nature in its pure crystallized form but always as the iodide with another compound, it was not seen until 1812. Bernard Courtois, a French Chemist, caught a glimpse of iodine condensing on the side of large vats used for cooking seaweed he was using to extract the gunpowder soda for Napoleon's army. Intermittently, the vats used for boiling the seaweed were cleaned of the residual debris after many boiling sessions. Courtois noticed one day, when he accidentally added too much acid, there were purple vapors rising from the mixture at the bottom. These vapors condensed into beautiful purple crystals on the sides of the cold vats. Courtois gathered some of the material and gave samples of it to one of the most prominent chemists in France, Gay-Lussac. Later Gay-Lussac went on to name the compound after the Greek meaning for violet colour and the French version of this was gradually changed to Iodine in English. This sequence of events led to one of the most significant medical advances of all time.

Iodine sources

Iodine-containing compounds are found in ashes of burnt seaweed, salty oil-well brines and Chilean Saltpetre, which is Sodium iodate. (Na IO3). Iodine is extracted in huge amounts by Japanese seaweed farming. Originally, during the formation of the earth, iodine dispersed throughout rock formations. Much later ocean water, plants and animals also contained iodine in low amounts. It was abundant, however, in seaweeds. Because of iodine's low concentrations everywhere on the planet, almost without exception single celled micro-organisms did not use iodine for any purpose. Erosion of the rocks by rain, glaciers, ice age, and later melting, leeched these small amounts of iodine out of the soil and rocks and washed them into the oceans where concentrations of sea salt is so low it does not prevent goiter in humans.

Because rains containing iodine from the ocean, older soils seen in New Mexico, contain more iodine than younger soils. Also, soil areas stripped of topsoil by glaciers, such as the North American Great Lakes regions, became endemic goiter areas. Dogs, humans, fish and likely other animals were iodine deficient and had goiters. In humans, goiter incidence fell below 1% because of iodine salt supplementation, but fish of the great lakes still show goiter formation. Iodine replacement of soil depletion by rain is a slow process. Soils depleted of iodine by the last ice age are still deficient in iodine. **Figure 1**

Iodine's role in antisepsis

Jean Lugol, a Paris physician, discovered iodine was made more soluble in water by potassium iodide. This discovery allowed the antiseptic properties of iodine solutions to be exploited, one century later, to sterilize every surface and material in hospitals. Its antiseptic potency and safety were never equaled or surpassed, as dilute iodine solutions kill all single celled organisms such as bacteria, viruses, fungi and protozoa. Not only are Lugol's solutions bactericidal at high dilutions, like 1/170,000, for standard pathogens such as Staphylococcus, but also iodine has the broadest range of action, fewest side effects and no development of bacterial resistance.

The most significant evolutionary event for eukaryote (nucleated cells organisms), including humans, occurred when seaweeds concentrated iodine. From this process came multicellular organisms, vertebrates and humans. Because iodine was not available in significant concentrations for much of evolution, single celled organisms blissfully reproduced themselves with structural membrane proteins having the amino acid tyrosine or histidine exposed to the surrounding medium or extra-cellular fluids. Iodine kills single celled organisms by combining with these same two amino acids. All single celled organisms showing tyrosine (tyrosyl) linkages exposed in the membrane proteins are killed by this simple chemical reaction that denatures proteins and kills the cells. **Figure 2**

Goitre and Iodine deficiency

Not long after the discovery of iodine, and without knowing iodine was the active ingredient of burnt seaweed, a physician in Geneva, Switzerland named Jean Francois Coindet announced that burnt ash of seaweed shrank thyroid enlargements (goiter). Coindet's findings hit the world by storm. For the first time in the history of medicine there was a specific treatment for a specific disease.

Because iodine deficiency can occur anywhere in the world and iodine is a sine qua non of fetal brain development, lack of iodine during pregnancy is the leading cause of intellectual impairment in the world. The prevention of iodine deficiency damage done to infants is the most important achievable international health goal.

When iodine intake is low, both humans and animals will develop thyroid gland enlargement to maintain thyroid function. In endemically iodine deficient areas, people show a wide variation in the pathology and clinical symptoms. The worst neurological damage results in cretinism. To emphasize the point, adequate iodine supplementation to the mother— before conception results in a normal baby. **Figure 3**

Iodized salt reduces goiters, mental retardation and eliminates cretinism. Clinically obvious goiters disappeared rapidly within the first generation. Iodine deficiency effects on thyroid cancer takes many years or generations. Before iodized salt more malignant cancers of the thyroid predominated thyroid pathology specimens, but after decades of iodine supplementation more benign forms of thyroid cancer occur. If iodine intake rose further, in time, the less malignant cancers would also disappear and theoretically at higher levels even hyperplasia (increase in the number of cells) would not occur.

The thrust of the thesis is that there are numerous benefits to raising the iodine intake to higher levels than current standards. But the early studies in the 1800s caused fear of iodine that made iodine supplementation as conservative as possible. So, the lowest dose of iodine daily preventing formation of goiter is the standard used world wide. Japan is extraordinary in that it has the highest daily intake of iodine and the lowest rates of cancer in the world in every organ except the stomach.

At the time of iodine's discovery, most of the world was iodine deficient. Therefore attempts at iodine supplementation met real problems of reactions to excess iodine. Some of the people, with Hashimoto's disease, became hypothyroid (low thyroid) because their thyroids could not handle the increased iodine intake. Autonomous nodules (working by themselves) in the thyroid of some people, took up excess iodine and made the patient hyperthyroid. These problems eventually stopped all iodine trials and resulted in a fear of iodine.

David Marine studied the goiters of dogs, fish and humans in the iodine deficient areas of the Great Lakes region. For preventing goiters, he found lower iodine doses more effective and that a year's supply of iodine could be given in a two-week period. In 1917, one hundred years after the discovery of iodine, Dr. David Marine and his associates solved the iodine supplementation problem. As a result, goiters in North America and Europe disappeared.

Iodine and the thyroid gland Figure 4

The basic unit of the thyroid gland is the follicle. The thyroid gland captures dietary iodine, synthesizes thyroid hormone from it, and stores thyroid hormone until it is needed. Colloid, the material in the center of the follicles, stores thyroid hormone in a large protein called thyroglobulin. Hydrolysis (digestion) of thyroglobulin releases thyroid hormone into the circulation in the form of thyroxine (T4) and triiodothyronine (T3).

Autoimmune thyroiditis

Besides goiters and thyroid cancers, autoimmune diseases of the thyroid are seen in iodine deficient regions. In the course of a minor illness, damaged thyroid cells dump their contents into the blood stream. Several proteins coming from the dead cells are foreign to the body immune system. The immune system having made antibodies to these proteins now attacks normal thyroid tissue causing inflammation and further death of thyroid gland cells. This mechanism is responsible for the initiation of Hashimoto's disease, Graves' disease and Exophthalmos behind the eyes.

Iodine in evolution

Iodine is widely dispersed in rocks but the concentration is extremely low and even the leeching of iodine from soil over ages did not raise the ocean's concentration significantly. Early development of single celled organisms such as bacteria, fungi, viruses, and protozoa arose without iodine. The earliest signs of iodine use are in diatoms (algae), but significant iodine concentration occurred in seaweeds.

Seaweed was the first to start capturing iodine from ocean water by a membrane transport mechanism that today still concentrates iodine to 20,000 times the ocean's concentration. What is not generally appreciated and perhaps not thought of in this light, was that the high concentrations of iodine in seaweed, whether the seaweed was dead or alive, gave birth to a brand new environment chemically different from the rest of the planet up to that time. This was the world of high iodine.

Never before had such an environment been created. For the first time there were no bacteria, fungi, viruses, or protozoa present. Archea are a different form of bacteria capable of growing in harsh environments and might have been the type of organism to colonize this niche. However, any new micro-organism trying to grow here would be under the influence of iodine and thyroxine.

Thyroxine (T4)

As iodination of almost any large protein results in the formation of thyroxine (T4), new cells colonizing the world of iodine would also contain thyroxine. So thyroxine formed from either intracellular proteins in the new cells or externally from cytoplasmic seaweed proteins. The genome and DNA of the new cell was in direct contact with iodine and thyroxine in the early stages of the formation of these new bacteria. At this crucial stage of formation thyroid hormone receptors formed in the cells and attached themselves to the DNA. Logically thyroxine took over control DNA or genome at this ancient time.

Formation of a nucleus

While thyroxine took control of the genome through thyroid hormone receptors, acidic iodine in the cytoplasm was attracting basic proteins. If this new cell attempted to enter the ocean, the high salt content of the ocean made it hypertonic to the cell and caused dehydration of the cell. The result would a condensed ball of chromatin, DNA and basic proteins. This bundle of chromatin and basic proteins now formed the first nucleus of a eukaryote (nucleated) cells, and it was important that this new nucleus was controlled by thyroxine. **Figure 6,7,8**

Following normal patterns of symbiosis this chromatin-containing nucleus ended up inside another new cell. Iodine within the cytoplasm of this cell provided a constant intracellular supply of thyroxine to control the DNA in the newly formed nucleus. Iodinated large proteins form thyroxine within their structure and have all the physiological potency for curing hypothyrodism as any currently used medications. Hence we now have a thyroxine run cell through DNA thyroxine receptors, a cellular membrane, a nucleus and an intracellular source of thyroxine.

If the latest development in the cells attempts to enter the ocean outside, again the cytoplasm of the cell collapses around the nucleus forming a double membrane. The collapsed cell becomes the cellular rough endoplasmic reticulum.

Energy producing Archea or bacteria formed in this high iodine environment would also have genomes and DNA responsive to thyroxine and tolerant of iodine. This energy producing cell likely was engulfed by the new nucleated cell and symbiotically incorporated into the cells as mitochondria. Now the nuclear DNA and the mitochondrial DNA were under thyroxine control. With identical thyroxine control, coordinated action between two cells led to a two-celled organism. Now, multicellular organisms prepared themselves for new attempts at leaving the seaweed and entering the ocean. But the rules of existence now demanded adequate iodine outside the cell and thyroxine inside. An iodine capturing mechanism such as the transport of iodine in seaweed was needed to extract iodine from the ocean.

Distribution of Iodine to other sites in the body

Dietary iodine is absorbed in the form of iodide into the blood stream where the thyroid captures iodine by a transport system similar to the one in seaweed. Also the salivary gland, breast, stomach and other tissues take up iodine out of the blood so their secretions have iodine levels 30 times levels in serum. Radioactive tracing of iodine shows that much of the iodine goes to the thyroid gland, nasal secretions, gut, breast, stomach, bone and in the extra-cellular fluids and connective tissue of almost all organs. Iodine can be found everywhere, for example, iodine appears in the cervical mucus within two minutes after injection. In evolution the gut served as the source of iodine before the thyroid gland appeared and now the gut serves as a reservoir of iodine for immediate needs of the body.

Iodine functions in the body.

The main function of the iodine is synthesis, storage and secretion of thyroid hormone. What iodine is left over is taken up in other tissues especially extra-cellular fluids and excreted in the urine. From extra-cellular fluids iodine travels in the lymphatics and re-enters the blood stream via the main lymphatic channel, the thoracic duct. In the 1960s it was established that if the daily dose of iodine was increased to over 2-3 mg of iodine per day, within two weeks, the thyroid became saturated and no longer took up iodine in significant amounts. So a normal person who raised their daily dose of iodine above, say 3 mgs, within two weeks their thyroid will almost completely stop taking up iodine as it becomes saturated, but more important to the body, all of the dietary iodine now went to perform other body functions.

Proposed other functions of iodine Figure 9.

The gradual sequence of changes from a slight abnormality, to slight changes in shape, size and intracellular structure, to a cancerous cell is a slow process that often takes many years. No effective immune system mechanism has been uncovered biochemically that removes abnormal non-cancerous forms of cells. As far as we can see, the immune system is not even good at recognizing single cancerous cells.

Relationship between bacteria and apoptosis

Many cells of the body are programmed to die. The natural death of cells on a regular and predictable schedule is called apoptosis. For example, mucus cells secreted into the stomach cavity have a life expectancy of 2-3 days. When we examine the location of iodine we see that there is abundant iodine at the sites in the body where apoptosis is active. It is now, we need to remember iodine's broad antiseptic action on single celled organisms. With such a mechanism for killing single cells in place, nature has the habit of utilizing such important mechanisms repeatedly. Such a simple chemical reaction between iodine and a tyrosine or histidine molecule on surface proteins is likely to be garnered by the new nucleated (eukaryote) cells. What better way than to use it to kill abnormal cells.. It could be that the outer membrane of eukaryote cells has hidden tyrosine or histidine molecule that are exposed by stretching of the membrane or exposed by just a change in the characteristics of the cell. By what we understand the iodine in the extra-cellular fluid would react with exposed tyrosine molecules and kill the cell in a manner similar to that of killing bacteria. Iodine then becomes the surveillance mechanism for abnormal cells in the body.

In areas of the body, where many cells die, there is always an endless source of iodine. The secretions into the nasal passages and lumen of the stomach come to mind as having both a high death rate and an endless supply of iodine. All the sites in the body of high apoptosis find iodine in plentiful supply. This mechanism then is for normal cells, so we suggest iodine does the same to abnormal cells developing in the body. Not only is iodine an antiseptic against bacteria when catgut for suturing is used on patients it also is an anticancer agent. It also will inhibit seeding during abdominal surgery for cancer.

Iodine excretion in the urine.

Iodine has an unusual excretion pattern in the urine. There are no re-absorption mechanisms or preservation mechanisms in the urinary tract to keep this element from excretion in the urine and hence loss from the body. If we acknowledge now that iodine is the trigger mechanism for apoptosis then it is imperative that a constant source of iodine in the urine be available. If the body was capable, and it is not, of holding the iodine inside and therefore allowing urine with no iodine to flow through the renal system then theoretically the renal system would be deprived of iodine. This would immediately lead to abnormal cells and cancer. A brief search of the literature reveals Australian workers found iodine caused apoptosis in a dose related fashion selectively in their tissue culture system.

Migration studies on Japanese

When Japanese women move to North America, descendants who consume a Westernized diet rapidly start to acquire cancer rates which are similar to those of North America. These studies suggest there is a dietary factor in the causation of breast cancer. It has been postulated that it is due to the Westernized diet. In fact this is true. The Western diet is nowhere near the levels needed to saturate the thyroid. An increase of at least 10 times would be helpful but more effective would be levels that are comparable to the Japanese.

Other functions of iodine in the stomach

From the work of Heneine and Heneine we can propose more protective functions for iodine in the lumen of the stomach. They showed clearly, the simple chemical reaction iodinating tyrosine and histidine in vitro deactivated biological poisons such as snake poisons. This must be one of the important actions of iodine. Coincidently, there is a well-known folk-ore that the best antidote for food poisoning, if it is suspected, is Lugol's solution of iodine swallowed in a glass of water. Chemically, also, we know iodine deactivates chemical toxins.

Antisepsis in the stomach

Iodine must have antiseptic activity in the stomach. The Japanese high incidence of helicobacter pylori in their stomachs relates to their high incidence of stomach cancer. This paradox, and exception to the iodine apoptosis mechanism model is likely related to nitrates and is discussed in the section on cancer. But the normal activity of iodine must be to protect the stomach from pathogenic organisms.

Iodine and food allergies

The Brazilian group found large foreign proteins were made non-allergic by reactions with iodine. That seems to explain an old observation seen in the study of iodine in the thoracic duct of dogs. It was found that the concentration of iodine in the thoracic duct, which is draining the stomach and intestines, is about five times the level in the serum. But if milk was fed to the dogs the thoracic duct iodine content went up by 20-30 times. This implies that iodine does in fact coat the foreign proteins like milk and allows them to enter the circulation protected from the immune system attack on a foreign protein.

Iodine and autoimmune disorders

Autoimmune diseases are related to a minor damage to the cells of the thyroid gland, pancreas and others. When the dead cells dump their contents into the blood stream, some of these proteins are foreign to the body, consequently, the immune system makes antibodies to them. These antibodies can go on to attack normal tissues. It seems logical that if there was enough iodine in the blood stream the discarded proteins from dead cells will be made non-allergic by a coating of iodine. Thus the origin of autoimmune diseases could relate to inadequate circulating iodine at the time of the illness, which caused the damage.

Iodine's ability to dissolve into lipids

The vague link between fat intake and breast cancer might be related to fat removing a micronutrient. One of the ways to measure the number of double bonds in fat is to measure the amount of iodine 100 grams of fat would take up. This was called the iodine number or value. The most unsaturated fat has the highest iodine value. But at the same time early experiments in the first half of the century showed puppies fed a high fat diet developed goiters. This suggests dietary fat removes iodine from the diet. It may be iodine protects double bonds while they are being transported to the sites where they are needed such a blood vessels and synaptic membranes of the central nervous system discussed by Crawford and Marsh.

Iodine in cervical secretions

Radioactive iodine injected intravenously shows up in the cervical mucosal secretions within two minutes. If we know that the iodine is antiviral, antibacterial and gets rid of abnormal cells then it follows that those with an adequate diet of iodine daily will have a lower incidence of cervical dysplasia or cancer of the cervix as seen in the Japanese.

Iodine and pregnancies

We know that during pregnancy the placenta captures iodine to the point of raising the levels in the fetal circulation to five times the mother's level. As there are a huge number of cells dying by apoptosis during fetal growth, it is not unreasonable to postulate that iodine is of importance to the fetal development. The brain has more apoptosis going on during development than most other organs, so it follows low iodine may cause abnormal brain development

Iodine and the developing fetus

Morreale de Escobar et al. have demonstrated that early fetal development is partly under the guidance of maternal thyroid hormones that have crossed the placenta. What has not yet seemed to be entertained is could the primitive cells at the beginning of fetal development still have the ability to make thyroid hormone themselves for their own use as postulated in the early evolution of eukaryotes. In 1912 Guttanch showed thyroid hormones would change a tadpole into a frog. This metamorphosis is complex at all levels. The tails dissolve away, legs are developed on the side, lungs are changed over to air breathing and liver, without any detectable change in the DNA or cellular morphology, changes over biochemical mechanisms from an ocean water animal to a land animal. Although the effects of thyroid hormone appear to be systemic in the tadpole, in fact, thyroid hormone is affecting each cell individually. But more importantly, if the thyroid gland is removed and iodine is given in any form— injection, orally or in the bathing solution— the metamorphosis will carry along at the same rate as if thyroid hormone was present. This suggests the ability of tadpoles to synthesize thyroid hormone from iodine alone is retained inside every cell. If this phenomena of intracellular synthesis of thyroxine has been carried over from the first days of eukaryote genesis, why wouldn't human fetal development also in its early stages be dependent on thyroxine manufactured from iodine within the cell? That would mean that, as has been found in developing countries, the only factor which completely eliminates cretinism, hypothyroidism in the fetus, and mental retardation is iodine given by any means as long as it is adequate —before conception.

Japanese women low birth defects and perinatal mortality?

Japanese women, who consume the highest amounts of iodine per woman in the world, have the lowest rate of stillbirth and peri- natal and infant mortality in the world. Their multi-century experience and knowledge was accumulated by Japanese mothers for many generations. But also among the folklore of Japanese mothers is the interesting concept that seaweed will prevent cancer.

Figure 1

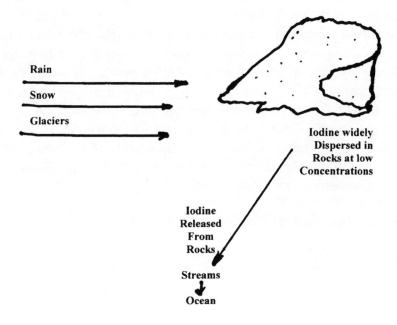

Rain

Snow

Glaciers

Iodine widely
Dispersed in
Rocks at low
Concentrations

Iodine
Released
From
Rocks

Streams

Ocean

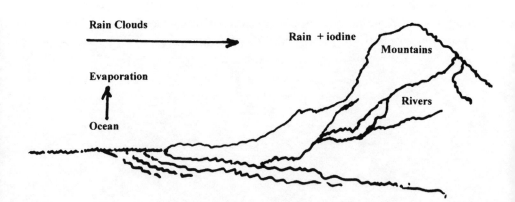

Rain Clouds

Rain + iodine

Mountains

Evaporation

Rivers

Ocean

Figure 2

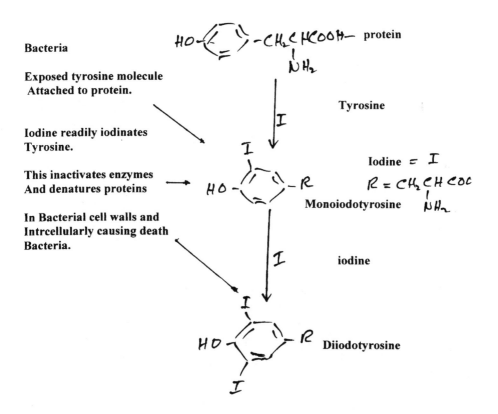

Bacteria

**Exposed tyrosine molecule
Attached to protein.**

**Iodine readily iodinates
Tyrosine.**

**This inactivates enzymes
And denatures proteins**

**In Bacterial cell walls and
Intrcellularly causing death
Bacteria.**

Figure 3

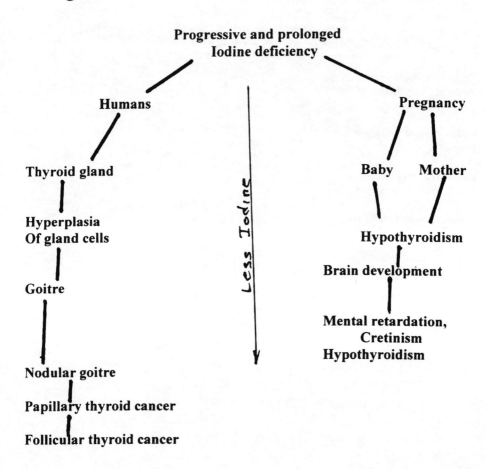

Figure 4

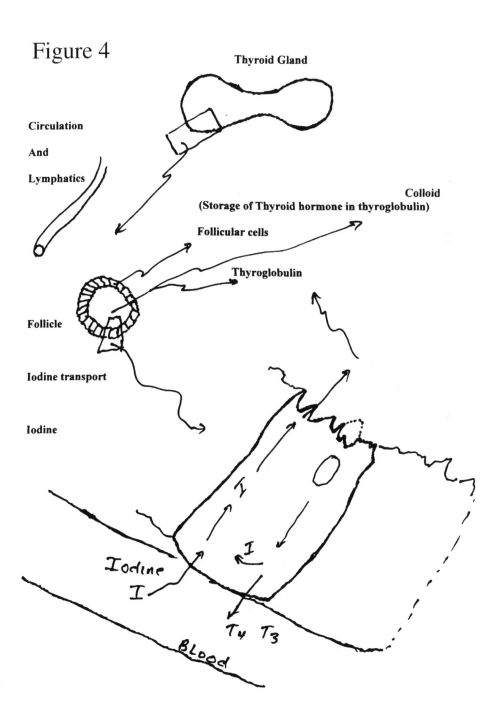

Thyroid Gland

Circulation

And

Lymphatics

Colloid
(Storage of Thyroid hormone in thyroglobulin)

Follicular cells

Thyroglobulin

Follicle

Iodine transport

Iodine

Iodine
I

I

I

T_4 T_3

Blood

World of high iodne

Figure 5

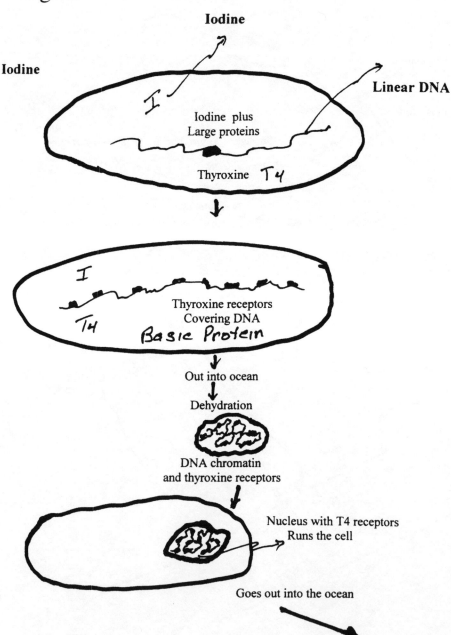

Iodine

Iodine

Linear DNA

Iodine plus
Large proteins

Thyroxine T4

Thyroxine receptors
Covering DNA
Basic Protein

Out into ocean

Dehydration

DNA chromatin
and thyroxine receptors

Nucleus with T4 receptors
Runs the cell

Goes out into the ocean

Figure 6

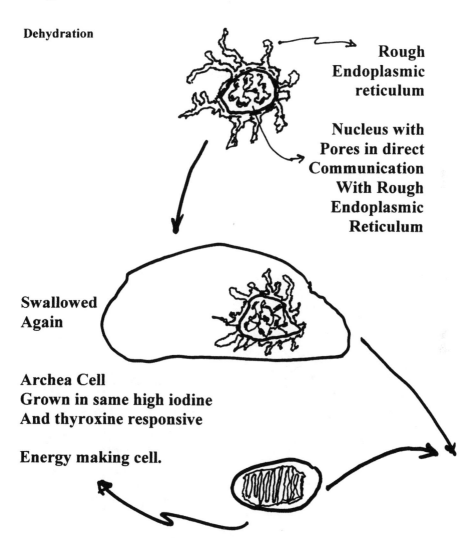

Dehydration

Rough
Endoplasmic
reticulum

Nucleus with
Pores in direct
Communication
With Rough
Endoplasmic
Reticulum

Swallowed
Again

Archea Cell
Grown in same high iodine
And thyroxine responsive

Energy making cell.

Figure 7

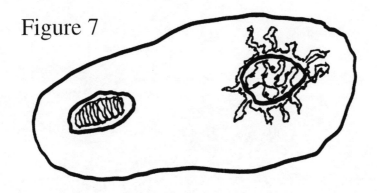

Eukaryote cell (nucleated cell)
Ready to join with other cells
Will take in more organelles

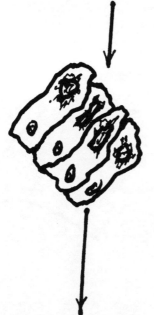

All cells have
Thyroxine receptors
On genome DNA
And
Mitochondrial DNA

Differentiation of multi-cell organisms

Figure 8

Proposed functions of iodine in human body

1. Used to make thyroid hormone in thyroid gland
2. Main body surveillance mechanism for abnormal cells in body.
3. Triggers Apoptosis (program death of cells) in normal cells and abnormal cells.
4. Detoxifies chemicals
5. Reacts with tyrosine and histidine to inactivate enzymes and denature proteins.
6. Antiseptic to bacteria, algae, fungi, viruses and protozoa.
7. Detoxifies biological toxins food poisoning, snake venoms etc.
8. Anti Allergic process. Makes external proteins non allergic
9. Anti autoimmune mechanism by making intracellular proteins spilled into blood non-allergic.
10. Protection of double bonds in lipids for delivery to cardiovascular system and synaptic membrances in brain and retina.
11. Fetal source of apoptitic mechanisms during development in fetus and breast-fed children.
12. Protection from apoptotic diseases such as Leukemia.
13. Possible initial source of thyroxine in early fetal development.
14. Antiseptic activity in stomach against helicobacter pylori.

Iodine References

1. Iodine and the brain (1988). New York: Plenum Press
2. Mechanisms of microbial disease (1989). Baltimore: Williams & Wilkins.
3. Hormones from molecules to disease (1990). New York: Hermann Publishers in Arts and Science, Chapman and Hall.
4. Thyroid disease (1990). New York: Raven Press.
5. Werner and Ingbar's The Thyroid (1991). (6 ed.) Philadelphia: J.B. Lippincott Company.
6. Williams textbook of endocrinology (1992). (Eigth ed.) Philadelphia: W.B. Saunders Co.
7. Endocrinology (1995). (Third ed.) (Vols. 1, 2 and 3) Philadelphia': W.B. Saunders Co.
8. Metamorphosis (1996). Toronto: Academic press.
9. Alberts, B., Bray, D., Lewis, J., Raff, M., Roberts, K., & Watson, J. D. (1989). Molecular biology of the cell. (Second ed.) New York: Garland Publishing, Inc.
10. Atkins, P. W. (1995). The periodic kingdom. New York: Basic Books A Division of Harper Collins Publishers.
11. Barnes, R. D. (1980). Invertebrate Zoology. (fourth ed.) Philadelphia: Saunders College/Holt, Rinehart and Winston.
12. Barrington, E. J. (1979). Invertebrate Structure and function. (Second ed.) Sunbury-on-Thames: Thomas Nelson and Sons Ltd.

13. Behrns, K. E., Schrum, L., & Que, F. G. (1999). Apoptosis: cell death by proteolytic scalpel. Surgery, 126, 463-468.

14. Benton, M. J. & Harper, D. A. (1997). Basic Palaeontology. Edinburgh Gate, England: Addison Wesley Longman.

15. Bergeron, C. (1995). Oxidative stress: its role in the pathogenesis of amyotrophic lateral sclerosis. Journal of the Neurological Sciences, 129 Suppl, 81-84.

16. Borow, D. J., Triplehorn, C. A., & Johnson, N. F. (1992). An introduction to the study of Insects. (Sixth ed.) New York: Saunders Colleg Publishing.

17. Braverman, L. E. (1994). Iodine and the thyroid: 33 years of study. Thyroid, 4, 351-356.

18. Braverman, L. E. (1998). Adequate iodine intake—the good far outweighs the bad [comment]. European Journal of Endocrinology, 139, 14-15.

19. Brock, T. D. & Madigan, M. T. (1991). Biology of Microorganisms. (Sixth ed.) Englewood Cliffs, New Jersey: Prentice Hall.

20. Brown-Grant, K. (1961). Extrathyroidal iodide concentrating mechanisms. Physiol Rev, 41, 189.

21. Campbell, N. A. (1990). Biology. (Second ed.) New York: The Benjamin/Cummings Publishing Company.

22. Carrol, B., Keosian, J., & Steinman, I. D. (1955). The mode of action of iodine on infectious agents. J Newark Beth Israel Hosp, 6, 129-140.

23. Cavalieri, R. R. (1997a). Iodine metabolism and thyroid physiology: current concepts. Thyroid, 7, 177-181.

24. Cavalieri, R. R. (1997b). Iodine metabolism and thyroid physiology: current concepts. Thyroid, 7, 177-181.

25. Cohn, I. J. (1967). Implantation in cancer of the colon. Surgery, Gynecology & Obstetrics, 124, 501-508.

26. Cohn, I. J. (1971). Cause and prevention of recurrence following surgery for colon cancer. Cancer, 28, 183-189.

27. Connolly, K. J. & Pharoah, P. O. (1981). Behavioural sequelae of fetal iodine deficiency. Progress in Clinical & Biological Research, 77, 383-391.

28. Davenport, H. W. Secretion of iodide by the gastric mucosa. Gastroenterology 1, 1055-1061. 1943.

29. Davidson, J. P., Reed, W. E., & David, P. M. (1997). Exploring Earth. Upper Saddle River, NJ.: Prentice Hall.

30. Dickhoff, W. W. & Darling, D. S. Evolution of thyroid function and its control in lower vertebrates. Amer Zool 23, 697-707. 1983.

31. Doolittle, W. F. Phylogenetic classification and the universal tree. Science 284, 2124-2128. 1999.

32. Dunn, J. T. (1993). Iodine supplementation and the prevention of cretinism. Annals of the New York Academy of Sciences, 678, 158-168.

33. Dunn, J. T. (1996). Seven deadly sins in confronting endemic iodine deficiency, and how to avoid them. Journal of Clinical Endocrinology & Metabolism, 81, 1332-1335.

34. Eales, J. G. (1997). Iodine metabolism and thyroid-related functions in organisms lacking thyroid follicles: are thyroid hormones also vitamins? Proceedings of the Society for Experimental Biology & Medicine, 214, 302-317.

35. Elmer, A. W. (1938). Iodine metabolism. London: Oxford University Press.

36. Faber, H. K. & Dong, L. (1953). Virucidal activity of some common surface antiseptics with special reference to poliomyelitis. Pediatrics, 12, 657.

37. Freshney, R. I. (1994). Culture of animal cells. New York: Wiley-Liss, A John Wiley & Sons, Inc. Publication.

38. Futuyma, D. J. (1998). Evolutionary Biology. (third ed.) Sunderland, Massachusetts: Sinaueer Associates,Inc.

39. Galton, V. A., Cohen, J. S., & Munck, K. (1982). T4 5'-monodeiodinase: The acquisition and significance of this enzyme system in the developing Rana Catesbeiana Tadpole. In T.Inui (Ed.), Phylogenetic aspects of thyroid hormone action (pp. 75-90). Tokyo: Center of acadamic publications Japan.

40. Gershenfeld, L. (1977a). Iodine. In S.S.Block (Ed.), Disinfection, Sterilization and Preservation (2 ed., pp. 196-218). Philadelphia: Lea & Febiger.

41. Gershenfeld, L. (1977b). Iodine. In S.S.Block (Ed.), Disinfection, Sterilization and Preservation (2nd ed., pp. 196-218). Philadelphia: Les & Febiger.
42. Gilbert, S. F. (1997). Developmental Biology. (Fifth ed.) Sunderland, Massachusetts: Sinauer Associates, Inc.
43. Globel, B., Globel, H., & Andres, C. (1985). The risk of hyperthyroidism following an increase in the supply of iodine. Journal of Hospital Infection, 6 Suppl A, 201-204.
44. Gubareff, N. & Suntzeff, V. (1962). Preliminary report on application of iodine in prevention of surgical dissemination of viable malignant cells. J Surg Res, 2, 144
45. Hays, M. T. Comparmental models for human iodide metabolism. Math Biosciences 72, 317-335. 1984.
46. Heneine, I. F. & Heneine, L. G. (1998). Stepwise iodination. A general procedure for detoxification of proteins suitable for vaccine development and antiserum production [comment]. Biologicals, 26, 25-32.
47. Herter, F. P. & Sbuelz, B. (1966). Inhibition of tumor growth by iodized catgut. Journal of Surgical Research, 6, 393-396.
48. Hetzel, B. S. (1989). The story of iodine deficiecy An international challange in nutrition. Oxford New York Tokyo: Oxford University Press.
49. Hofstadter, F. (1980). Frequency and morphology of malignant tumours of the thyroid before and after the introduction of iodine-prophylaxis. Virchows Archiv.A, Pathological Anatomy & Histology, 385, 263-270.
50. Hurrell, R. F. (1997). Bioavailability of iodine. European Journal of Clinical Nutrition, 51 Suppl 1, S9-12.
51. Jalayer, T. & Askari, I. (1966). A study of the effect of aqueous iodine on hydatid cysts in vitro and in vivo. Annals of Tropical Medicine & Parasitology, 60, 169-171.
52. Kardon, K. V. (1997). Vertebrates comparative anatomy, function, evolution. New York: WCB McGraw-Hill.
53. Kelly, F. C. Iodine in medicine and pharmacy since its discovery—1811-1961. Proc R Soc Med 54, 831-836. 1961.
54. Knaysi, G. (1932). The toxicity of iodine for the cells of Mycobacterium tuberculosis. J Infect Dis, 50, 253-260.

55. Konno, N., Yuri, K., Miura, K., Kumagai, M., & Murakami, S. (1993). Clinical evaluation of the iodide/creatinine ratio of casual urine samples as an index of daily iodide excretion in a population study. Endocrine Journal, 40, 163-169.

56. Lamberg, B. A. (1993). Iodine deficiency disorders and endemic goitre. [Review] [47 refs]. European Journal of Clinical Nutrition, 47, 1-8.

57. Lamberg, B. A., Haikonen, M., Hintze, G., Honkapohja, H., Hiltunen, R., & Pulli, K. (1970). Regression of endemic goitre and of changes in iodine metabolism during 10-15 years in the east of Finland. The role of iodine prophylaxis. Hormones, 1, 80-95.

58. Lee, K., Bradley, R., Dwyer, J., Lee, S. L., & ' (1999). Too much or too little: The implication of current Iodine intake in the United States. Nutrition Reviews, 57, 177-181.

59. Lee, S. M., Lewis, J., Buss, D. H., Holcombe, G. D., & Lawrence, P. R. Iodine in British foods and diets. B J of Nutrition 72, 435-446. 1994.

60. Levinton, J. S. (1995). Marine Biology, function, biodiversity, ecology. New York: Oxford University Press.

61. Lodish, H., Berk, A., Zipursky, S. L., Matsudaira, P., Baltimore, D., & Darnell, J. (1999). Molecular Cell Biology. New York: W.H.Freeman and Company.

62. Lynn, W. G. & Wachowski, H. E. (1951). Quart.Rev.Biol., 26, 123.

63. Lyons, A. S. & Petrucelli, R. J. (1987). Medicine an Illustraed History. New York: Abradale Press Harry N. Abrams, Inc., Publishers.

64. Maberly, G. F. (1994). Iodine deficiency disorders: contemporary scientific issues. Journal of Nutrition, 124, 1473S-1478S.

65. MacMahon, B., Cole, P., Lin, T. M., Lowe, C. R., Mirra, A. P., Ravnihar, B., Salber, E. J., Valaoras, V. G., & Yuasa, S. Age at first birth and breast cancer risk. Bull Wld Hlth Org. 43, 209-221. 1970.

66. Madigan, M. T., Martinko, J. M., & Parker, J. A. (1997). Brock Biology of microorganisms. (Eigth ed.) Upper Saddle River,NJ O7458: Prentice Hall.

67. Mizukami, Y., Michigishi, T., Nonomura, A., Hashimoto, T., Tonami, N., Matsubara, F., & Takazakura, E. (1993). Iodine-induced hypothyroidism: A clinical and histological study of 28 patients. J of Clinical Endocrinology and Metabolism, 76, 466-471.

68. Morreale de Escobar, G. & et al (1991). Maternal thyroid hormones during pregnancy: effects on the fetus in congenital hypothyroidism and in iodine deficiency. Adv Exp Med Biol, 299, 133-156.

69. Mutvei, A., Husman, B., Andersson, G., & Nelson, B. D. (1989). Thyroid hormone and not growth hormone is the principle regulator of mammalian mitochondrial biogenesis. Acta Endocrinol.(Copenh.), 121, 223-228.

70. Oddie, T. H. & et al (1970). Iodine intake in the United States: a reassessment. J Clin Endocr Metab, 30, 659-665.

71. Pechenik, J. A. (1996). Biololgy of Invertebrates. (Third ed.) Toronto: Wm. C. Brown Publishers.

72. Pennington, J. A. (1990). A review of iodine toxicity reports. J.Am.Diet.Assoc., 90, 1571-1581.

73. Porter, R. (1997). Greatest benefit to mankind A Medical history of humanity. New York: W.W. Norton & Company.

74. Potter, J. D., McMichael, A. J., & Hetzel, B. S. (1979). Iodization and thyroid status in relation to stillbirths and congenital anomalies. International Journal of Epidemiology, 8, 137-144.

75. Preux, P. M., Couratier, P., Boutros-Toni, F., Salle, J. Y., Tabaraud, F., Bernet-Bernady, P., Vallat, J. M., & Dumas, M. (1996). Survival prediction in sporadic amyotrophic lateral sclerosis. Age and clinical form at onset are independent risk factors. Neuroepidemiology, 15, 153-160.

76. Raven, P. H., Evert, R. F., & Eichhorn, S. E. (1999). Biology of Plants. (Sixth ed.) New York: W.H. Freeman and Company.

77. Reddish, G. F. (1957). <u>Antiseptics, disinfectants fungicides and chemical and physical sterilization.</u> Philadelphia: Lea & FebigerHa.
78. Riggs, J. E., Schochet, S. S. J., & Gutmann, L. (1984). Benign focal amyotrophy. Variant of chronic spinal muscular atrophy. <u>Archives of Neurology, 41,</u> 678-679.
79. Saikumar, P., Dong, Z., Mikhailov, V., Denton, M., Weinberg, J. M., & Venkataraman, M. (1999). Apoptosis: Definition, mechanisms, and relevance to disease. <u>American Jounal of Medicine, 107,</u> 489-506.
80. Salter, W. T. Fluctuations in body iodine. Physiol Rev 20, 345-376. 1940.
81. Salter, W. T. (1951). <u>Endocrine function of iodine.</u> (1st ed.) Cambridge, Mass.: Harvard.
82. Schaller, R. T. & et al. (1966). Development of carcinoma of the thyroid in iodine-deficient mice. <u>Cancer, 19,</u> 1063-1080.
83. Shaw, T. I. Mechanism of iodide accumulation by the brown seaweed Laminaria digitata I.Uptake of I131. Proc Roy Soc (London) B 150, 356-371. 1959.
84. Smerdely, P., Pitsiavas, V., & Boyages, S. C. (1993). Evidence that the inhibitory effects of iodide on thyroid cell proliferation are due to arrest of the cell cycle at G0G1 adn G2M phases. <u>Endocrinology, 133,</u> 2881-2888.
85. Stanbury, J. B. (1992). Iodine and human development. [Review] [33 refs]. <u>Medical Anthropology, 13,</u> 413-423.
86. Stowe, C. M. (1981). Iodine, iodides, and iodism. <u>Journal of the American Veterinary Medical Association, 179,</u> 334-336.
87. Stryer, L. (1988). <u>Biochemistry.</u> (Third ed.) New York: W.H. Freeman and Company.
88. Thomson, C. D., Colls, A. J., Conaglen, J. V., Macormack, M., Stiles, M., & Mann, J. (1997). Iodine status of New Zealand residents as assessed by urinary iodide excretion and thyroid hormones. <u>British Journal of Nutrition, 78,</u> 901-912.

89. Thorpe-Beeston, J. G. & Nicolaides, K. H. (1996). Maternal and fetal thyroid function in pregnancy. New York: The Parthenon Publishing Group.

90. Turner, G. D. (1955). General Endocrinology. (2 ed.) Philadelphia: W.B. Saunders Company.

91. Vagenakis, A. G. (1990). Effects of iodides: clinical studies. Thyroid, 1, 59-63.

92. Vagenakis, A. G. & et al. (1973). Control of thyroid hormone secretion in normal subjects receiving iodides. Journal of Clinical Investigation, 52, 528-532.

93. Vernick, J. J. & Hoppe, E. T. (1966). The value of iodine compounds in the experimental treatment of wounds inoculated with cancer cells. Surgery, 59, 278-281.

94. Watson, J. D., Hopkins, N. H., Roberts, J. W., Steitz, J. A., & Weiner, A. M. (1988). Molecular Biology of the gene. (Forth ed.) Don Mills, Ontario: The Benjamin/Cummings Publishing Company Inc.

95. Wayne, E. J., Koutras, D. A., & Alexander, W. D. (1964). Clinical aspects of iodine metabolism. Philadelphia: F.A. David Company.

96. Wiseman, R. A. (2000). Breast cancer hypothesis: a single cause for the majority of cases. J Epidemiol Community Health, 54, 851-858.

97. Woese, C. The universal ancestor. Proc Natl Acad Sci 95, 6854-6859. 1998.

98. Wolfe, S. L. (1995a). An introduction to cell and molecular biology. New York: Wadsworth Publishing Company and International Thomson Publishing Company.

99. Wolfe, S. L. (1995b). Cell and Molecular Biology. New York: Wadsworth Publishing Co An international Thomson Publishing Co.

100. Wooten, W. L. & et al. (1980). The effect of thyroid hormone on mitochondrial biogenesis and cellular hyperplasia. J Bioenerg Biomembr, 12, 1-12.

101. Wynder, E. L. The epidemiology of large bowel cancer. Cancer Res 35, 3388-3394. 1975.

Thyroid gland and thyroid hormone.

 The new single cell, that developed in the high iodine environment was totally independent, except for a need for iodine, from the environment. It could not only synthesize its own thyroid hormone but also controlled the genome through thyroid hormone and its receptors to run cellular function and metabolism. In this type of micro-organism the cells would all have been iodine tolerant, meaning they would not have exposed amino acids of tyrosine or histidine. The place for this new world of iodine and thyroxine to have started was likely in some way related to seaweed. This was the planet's first source of almost unlimited quantities of iodine. As iodination of proteins is a simple easy and predictable chemical reaction, which automatically produces thyroxine within the protein, so intracellular iodination of proteins likely was an original source of thyroxine to these early developing cells. These cells did not need to have an outside source of thyroxine.

   Through a series of events to do with attempts of the organism to leave the environment for the ocean led to hypertonic (dehydrating) solutions sucking all the water out of the new cells. This collapsed the basic proteins and linear DNA now covered with thyroid hormone receptors into what is now called the nucleus.

   A further similar chain of events likely led to the present rough endoplasmic reticulum. Energy production of these cells in this new environment developed with thyroid hormone receptors on their DNA, iodine tolerance and likely then joined the new nucleated cells symbiotically as mitochondria. From here, with a few more organelle acquisitions, the cells were now ready to cooperate with each other under the same control by thyroxine. Multicellular organisms were now possible. But in order to be able to move out of the seaweed high iodine environment to the ocean outside there would need to be protective mechanisms developed from the high salt content of the ocean. The new multicellular organism could have adjusted its own internal salt concentration closer to that of the ocean to make the transition to the outside world easier. Once the multicellular organism was outside and could survive it was important that a source of iodine be available and a mechanism for capturing it for the organism.

From here there must have been a blossoming of the number of experimental animals but with an overall new type of control of the genome.

Soon, in evolutionary time, the precursor of the thyroid, the endostyle or thyroid-hormone-making-site in the pre-vertebrate animals arrived. This organ in the back of the pharynx of primitive pre-vertebrates excreted protein bound thyroxine into the gut and there it was hydrolysed, absorbed and delivered all over the body. Later in early vertebrates, at a site close by to where the endostyle was, the first thyroid gland follicles can be discerned. By then thyroid hormone was being secreted internally into the blood. At this point there was no brain, pituitary or hypothalamus control mechanisms to influence the thyroid function.

The thyroid hormone is the first endocrine hormone to arrive in evolution and it is the first to arrive during fetal life. But almost simultaneously with the development of the thyroid gland, the central nervous system started to develop since the nerve cells were assured of a constant supply of thyroxine and this in turn depended upon a constant supply of iodine.

Eartly and Leblond in their classic article on thyroid gland and its effects, showed thyroid gland hormone has a direct effect on activation of metabolism but that all other effects of pituitary hormones were thyroxine mediated. **Figure 9A and 9B** show two diagrams on the relationships of the thyroid axis from an anatomical and physiological viewpoint.

The diagram of the physiological functions of thyroid hormone shows thyroxine controls all endocrine organs which is what we would expect if the thyroid controls the genome and also was the first to arrive in evolution and in fetal development. This physiological role of thyroid hormone and all the other hormones through the pituitary fits with the thesis put forward here that thyroxine gained control of the genome early in evolution.

Later the brain evolved into our present system of the hypothalamic-pituitary-thyroid system giving the hypothalamus overall control of the output of the thyroid gland. The pituitary feedback mechanism does not control the level of thyroid hormone controls maintenance of a steady level of thyroid hormone in the blood stream at all times. It appears that the most important event in the life of the pituitary thyroid system occurs at birth. Because the hypothalamus and the thyroid hormone control the body temperature at birth there is a serge in TSH (thyroid stimulating hormone)which greatly increases the thyroid hormone excreted into the blood at birth. This relates to metamorphic changes in the lungs and other systems as the baby switches over to air breathing.

After birth thyroid starts putting out a fairly constant supply of thyroid hormone for the rest of the human's life. The reserve of the thyroid gland to stress and its ability to respond appear related to adequate iodine intake before the age of puberty, which is the first real test of the thyroid's reserve abilities. In animals there are changes in the thyroid output at different seasonal and migratory events but in humans there are few events of this kind that seem to change the TSH significantly except some changes in pregnancy. But the stress on the thyroid can be detected and the size of the thyroid gland measured accurately by ultrasound. The thyroid enlargement from physiological stress found in areas of borderline low iodine intake, occur during adolescence, pregnancies and menopause. These enlargements are good indicators of borderline iodine supplementation indicating a degree of iodine deficiency, but at the same time this illustrates the increased needs for thyroid hormone during period of physiological stress during life.

Disturbance of the thyroid system relates to disease. A low output of thyroid hormone will not provide the cellular DNA with adequate thyroid hormone for proper maintenance. Also as each tissue controls its own thyroid metabolism the same levels of thyroid in the blood may not be adequate for the tissue adaptation mechanisms in another. There is no feedback system from individual tissues to tell the thyroid -TSH system to rise higher because one tissue is not getting enough. The brain seems to have the highest priority for maintenance of thyroid hormone levels. For example, if the patient has a thyroid gland that by lab tests is normal, but the patient has a low thyroid dependent depression, the depression will continue until somehow the level of thyroid hormone is raised above its current levels. The only way to do this is to supplement the patient's thyroid with thyroid hormone orally. The tendency nowadays to use antidepressants is still not diagnosing the underlying condition.

Although cretinism and related goiters have been noted through out all ages, it wasn't until the discovery of iodine that some progress, albeit very slow, was made in the understanding of the thyroid gland. But clinically the most historic document on thyroid occurred in 1888. This committee described a variable syndrome in persons whose thyroid had been removed or were suffering from a completely failed thyroid. To this was given the name myxedema to stand for the presence of a peculiar type of mucin that gathered in almost all the connective tissues of the body.

One of the characteristics of extreme low thyroid is to find this mucin in virtually every organ of the body, however this seems quite reasonable now if we understand cellular and organ control of the thyroid action at the intracellular level. Many physicians have pointed out that the intracellular control mechanisms are central to the control of thyroid hormone action. When we also know that there are receptors for thyroid hormones in the cell membrane, the cytosol (intracellular sap), the mitochondria and the nucleus, we begin to understand how important this thyroid control system is.

Treatments using thyroid preparations

One hundred and ten years ago Fox and MacKenzie showed that oral thyroid preparations made from sheep thyroid were effective treatments for hypothyroidism from which oral desiccated thyroid then became the standard therapy for 80 years. Almost unbelievable transformations took place when the raw or cooked thyroid was given to the patients. Moribund nearly dead patients who were totally incapable of functioning were returned to normal life over a few short weeks of treatment. However, with the thyroid treatment it was necessary to continue the patient's therapy for the rest of their lives. No useful consistent way to rehabilitate the thyroid gland back to normal function has been discovered.

By 1976 about half (52%) of the prescriptions written for thyroid hormone in the United States were for desiccated thyroid or other natural products. The best pharmacological authorities confirmed desiccated thyroid remains a remarkably clinically predictable and effective preparation which is well absorbed. The medical letter in 1973 maintained that desiccated thyroid had never been unreliable. The slight variations in the T3 levels mentioned by some are of little clinical significance. A large shipment to distributors in the Europe and the United States in 1963 of what was supposed to be desiccated thyroid turned out to be tablets that contained iodine but no thyroid hormone. This was a hoax. Goodman and Gilman. stated "This episode gave thyroid a bad name because several publications about the unreliability of thyroid appeared before the hoax was uncovered." (1970). This hoax is the only record of desiccated thyroid being unreliable.

Selected descriptions of Mild hypothyroidism

By the 1930s Dr. George Crile and his associates wrote one of the early textbooks on thyroid diseases summarizing 40 years of clinical experience with thyroid hormone. In it he also described a form of hypothyroidism, which was milder and not as easy to recognize as the standard myxedema, which was an extreme variation on the low thyroid syndrome.

Dr. George Crile and his associates described in detail the symptoms of what he called incipient hypothyroidism. He emphasized there are varying degrees of low thyroid disease, the milder grade producing less definite and more obscure symptoms. This, he says, is particularly true of the milder forms of thyroid deficiency. "The fact that specific diagnostic methods are lacking and that other diagnosis can be made, which apparently explain the symptoms, results in failure to recognize the underlying condition in many of these cases." (low thyroid).

He did say that mild hypothyroidism is not life or death to the patient or even serious disability, but still the fact remains that the well-being of many people could be improved if this condition were more frequently detected in its early stages.

"Incipient hypothyroidism occurs at all ages.

In children mild deficiency may be the cause of behavior problems, or of a mild degree of mental slowness, which often is not abnormal enough to be given much consideration. In children of this type startling results occasionally follow the administration of small doses of thyroid extract."

"At puberty and in the early teens diminished endurance and a tendency to anemia, nervous disorders, problems with menstrual cycle or digestive disturbances often are explained by a mild degree of hypothyroidism."

"Extreme physical and nervous exhaustion in young adults, the depressions of middle life, and aggravated symptoms of menopause maybe partially explained on the basis of low thyroid. Late symptoms which simulate senile changes frequently are distinctly improved by the administration of thyroid extract."

"In review the body systems we find each may be affected by this disorder which is quite variable. Nervous disorders, such as headaches, neurasthenia, mild psychic disturbances, especially affective disorders (depression), fears, anxieties, poor memory, and difficult concentration are frequently seen."

"Circulation symptoms are referred chiefly to the heart and are caused by myocardial degeneration. Hypothyroidism predisposes to premature arteriosclerosis."

"Gastrointestinal symptoms are extremely common. Anorexia, distress after eating, belching of gas, vomiting, obstinate constipation, and occasional diarrhea."

"The menstrual function is especially susceptible to extremely mild thyroid deficiency and every type of disturbance may be seen from amenorrhea (no periods),to profuse menorrhagia (heavy bleeding), especially at menopause. That these disturbances may be due to hypothyroidism is evidenced by the improvement which results from the administration of thyroid extract in small doses."

"Sterility is a well-recognized result of this condition, and in all cases of sterility both the male and the female partner should be studied to see whether or not hypothyroidism is present in either."

"Joint symptoms, muscular aches and pains, skin disorders and many other minor disorders are reported to be the result of hypothyroidism."

"The ordinary effects of hypometabolism, obesity, depression, subnormal temperature, and susceptibility to cold, dry skin and brittle nails, and tendency to excessive drowsiness are of course frequently seen and one or more of the features usually are present in every case."

"The variations which may occur are surprising. Some patients show a very marked degree of nervous energy, some patients instead of being obese, are thin and emaciated and gain weight on thyroid medication, some complain of insomnia."

"When the diagnosis is in doubt a brief therapeutic trial of thyroid extract will not do any harm."

In 1942, August Werner's Endocrinology clinical application and treatment (Werner, 1942), has unique differences in his description of low thyroid conditions. Listed here are some of the symptoms he stated were related to low thyroid and would respond to thyroid therapy.

"Among these are subjective nervousness, poor emotional control, excitability, irritability with periods of depression at times. These people complain of easy fatigability. Although they may be energetic and have a desire to be active. They are easily exhausted. As the days work progresses they realize that it requires strong effort to finish. They cannot build up sufficient reserve energy to labour normally. This fatigue may be mental as well as physical, in which case there is an inability to think quickly and accurately."

"Occipital-cervical aching with radiation to the shoulders or intrascapular area is common. Also Rheumatoid pains may occur in various joints and parts of the body without evidence of inflammation."

"Blood cholesterol is often elevated. If the cholesterol is elevated, it is presumptive diagnosis of hypothyroidism. Finally a response to thyroid medication with return to normal of blood cholesterol makes the diagnosis definite."

It is worth remembering that all of these symptoms were treated with thyroid extract successfully. Most low thyroid problems could be diagnosed clinically with a careful history and physical examination. The only diagnostic tests worth doing at the time were the Basal Metabolic rate and the cholesterol.

Goal of treatment with thyroid

"The goal of treatment is freedom from symptoms with the minimum dose. We might say indeed instead of freedom from symptoms, merely maximum possible well-being".

Radioactive iodine?

In the 1940s two advances in thyroid treatment and study occurred. Radioactive isotope of iodine became available to study thyroid metabolism. Also anti-thyroid drugs that blocked the thyroid when it was overactive arrived. The result was a better understanding of thyroid physiology by the 1960s and new tests of thyroid function.

The two most important tests were the uptake of radioactive iodine in thyroid gland and the Protein Bound Iodine or PBI. Both tests were helpful but not full proof for diagnosis. There was much enthusiasm for the PBI as the only lab test needed to diagnose thyroid disease. Not so. Gradually it was found to be unreliable and was discarded in the late sixties for the arrival of the T4 and more importantly, the arrival of the TSH (thyroid stimulating hormone) in 1973. There were two articles one by Evered et al in the British Medical Journal in 1973 and JM Stock et al in the New England Journal of Medicine in 1974. The results of the TSH test in patients suggested treatment used clinically for 80 years previously was wrong. Patients could now be diagnosed and treated on the basis of the TSH. But the TSH test was so sensitive that all doses ended up being reduced by about two thirds.

There had been 80 years of clinical evaluation showing 200-400 micrograms of thyroxine was the normal dose to effectively make the patient feel well again and to return them back to normal. The equivalent amount of desiccated thyroid was 180-300 mgs. One third of those doses, such as 100 micrograms or less, now became the norm for treatment of low thyroid conditions after 1973. But there were two other effects. A trial of thyroid was no longer indicated because the TSH value dictated thyroid status. TSH was the diagnostic tool now.

Within two to three years the teaching changed completely. All of the signs and symptoms thought to be important in the past that were treated successfully by past physicians were now set aside. All that clinical experience was discarded. The students and endocrinologists in training were instructed to find another diagnosis for the common symptoms of low thyroid if the TSH was within the normal given guidelines. It was only rarely mentioned that there was no relation between the signs and symptoms of hypothyroidism and the value of the TSH. Meaning that a lab test was being monitored to treat the patients without any correlation to how the patient felt or their well-being.

Reasons for change

But this still does not tell us why treatment of low thyroid conditions changed, there had to be more reasons than stated above. The problem with treating low thyroid patients empirically with thyroid hormone was that there was another group of patients who were even more confusing. In order to sort this out it is necessary to go to the basic textbook of endocrinology in 1962 by Dr. Willams. At this time the hoax on the desiccated thyroid had not taken place so all treatments were with desiccated thyroid extract. In normal subjects thyroid medication in doses used then quickly turned the thyroid gland off as it was replaced by thyroid extract. So, up to certain levels of approximately 180 mgs (200 micrograms of thyroxine) there were no changes in the basal metabolic rate, the thyroid test of its time, the Protein Bound Iodine or clinical status. So any dose below this level was unlikely to make any difference to the patient.

Williams emphasized the need in most patients to get to a dose of 180 mgs before benefits would be felt. But, there were some puzzling patients who required up to 600 mgs to accomplish this effect. Williams said there is considerable difference in the metabolism or requirements of patients for thyroid hormone because of the common observation that certain patients can only tolerate 180 mgs daily whereas others can take 600 mgs with impunity. The reason for the variation in response of different patients was not solved.

In the group of patients who have normal blood tests but have symptoms of low thyroid Dr. Williams became frustrated. It is here that Dr. Williams expressed some concern about the effectiveness of all thyroid preparations in this group. He admitted some of these patients secure at least partial improvement of their symptoms with desiccated thyroid therapy. However the benefits often wane after a few months. With increased dosage new benefits are derived. This cycle may be repeated several times finally reaching large doses which to the patient and physician seems to no avail and this type of therapy was discontinued. There are some patients who never derive benefit from the therapy, while others continue to feel improved with a constant dosage of 120-180 mg. per day. The treatment of low thyroid conditions constantly required clinical assessment. Dr. Williams followed the policy of giving his patients a therapeutic trial with desiccated thyroid.

It is interesting that Dr. Williams used as an illustration of failure in some of these patients the Basal Metabolic rate on a patient with gradually increasing dosage of desiccated thyroid. The BMR gradually rose but even when the patient was up at 10 grains (600mgs) the effects of the desiccated thyroid worn off and the basal metabolic rate returned to normal. (about 800 micrograms of thyroxine) This patient illustrated some patients can take enormous doses that seem to wear off. This peculiar phenomenon led gradually to abandoning the clinical approach entirely and opting for a laboratory test, which would definitely tell the physician what to do without needing to assess the clinical status of the patient. The arrival of the two articles in 1973-4 started the inevitable process that resulted from clinicians just not knowing how to handle or explain these puzzling patients who were so tolerant of thyroid medication.

Sexual abuse or terror in childhood and thyroid hormone resistance.

One of the topics, rarely discussed in those days, was sexual or physical abuse in children. It is not surprising that the clinicians of that day did not enquire if the patients had severe childhood difficulties to the point of being frightened or terrorized for prolonged periods during their growing up years below the age of 12. Almost without exception, I have found patients who have a childhood history of abuse or prolonged fright of some sort react sluggishly or poorly to thyroid hormone. Many also give histories of puzzling reactions to other drugs.

These people appear to be pharmacologically (drug handling) different from normal people. Some people, as Dr. Williams stated, tolerate huge doses of thyroid hormone without any benefits or with only partial benefits. The confusion over this group of patients led the laboratory orientated physicians to take control of this confusing area with the TSH test and other related tests. It is possible that the receptor system for thyroid hormone and other drugs may be malleable under the age of 12, and adjustments to its sensitivity to thyroid hormone and likely other hormones enable them to better survive under frightening conditions. The receptor changes are permanent, as I have found people in this category over fifty. The treatment for these people needs to be re-evaluated. Sexually and physically abused people have had many counseling sessions which do not remove flash backs, fear and anxiety of their past, whereas thyroid medication over time appears to slowly adjust these well worn brain pathways of flashbacks, images and anxieties.

Thyroid seems to soften these images with time and the patient becomes more able to handle their past. It is as if the images are moved to the side —not cured — not eliminated—but not still right in their faces. With thyroid hormone therapy these people are more able to cope with the counseling they receive and to progress in dealing with their lives. It is not full proof but it is better than we have had for these unfortunate people. The thyroid hormone distinctly helps people's coping abilities. In terms of well-being, the person's coping mechanisms are a good clinical measure of the efficacy of treatment.

It is not generally appreciated that abused persons are wandering around in society unable to cope with daily life. Many are almost permanently semi-suicidal. Thyroid hormone in adequate doses seems to alleviate much of this.

So the confusion of Dr. Williams and the many who came after him about the variability of thyroid therapy was solely related to being unaware that many of these adults were the victims of some sort of childhood fear or abuse. In our present atmosphere of medical practice the laboratory results have effectively cut the patient off from empirical treatment with thyroid hormone therapeutically. Because of this many of these people are in trouble. In a milder expression of this problem, this phenomena has been analyzed by other workers.

Thyroid hormone resistance

Thyroid hormone resistance syndrome describes a clinical picture where there is variable tissue resistance to thyroid hormone. Since circulating thyroid hormone is normal, metabolism is through normal pathways and there is normal penetration of peripheral tissues, the defect must reside at the cellular site of thyroid hormone action. Thus, abnormalities of the receptor or defects at some post-receptor step in the expression of hormone action, is a plausible hypothesis. In terms of the abuse thesis, it is easier to postulate that the fear reaction of abused people below the age of 12 allows for some adaptive changes in the thyroid hormone receptor system likely as a biochemical survival tactic. They may be a large source of thyroid resistant people in the population.

Before the 1973-1974 change to laboratory diagnosis, the objective of treatment in all cases was to raise the thyroid dose up until the patient was in a state of well-being again. Within reason the individual patient response was more important than the dose or laboratory results. Therefore, the well-being and the return to normal function was the objective of treatment. Thyroid cancer and patients with goiters were given sub-toxic doses of thyroid hormone. That is, the dose was raised until the patient experienced some of the effects of too much thyroid such as sweating or racing heart then the dose was lowered just a bit below that dose. Thyroid hormone is a safe and effective therapeutic agent, which has not been used adequately since the 1973-1974 articles.

It is the purpose of this book to indicate some of the places where thyroid hormone can be used with an emphasis on the breast cancer patients. But, as we know, the well-being, constitutional health and coping abilities of patients is directly related to the effectiveness of thyroid hormone in the body of that individual. The one way to increase the well-being and constitution of a patient is with thyroid hormone.

Thyroid hormone is one of the greatest therapeutic agents of all time. It also is likely to be safer by far than much of the medicine we take today. Two medications came out of the last century (1800s), which are still used today - Aspirin and thyroid hormone. Aspirin overdoses have killed children regularly in the thousands since it first came out. Overdoses of thyroid have not been clinically significant and few are admitted to hospital. Few, if any, deaths have been reported of acute overdose.

Fear of thyroid hormone

In the process of supporting the laboratory process doctors have scared themselves and the public with the dangers of thyroid hormone. Before the 1973-1974 change, the normal dose of thyroid was three times the level seen now and there were no cases of fractures or osteoporosis ever reported in the previous 80 years. Yet, both are often mentioned by physicians, as dangers of using too much thyroid. Patients on doses used before 1973 felt better, energetic and motivated so they remained more active during all of their lives. This alone would be a factor in stopping osteoporosis. As all the osteoporosis questions came after the use of thyroxine came into vogue, it is not clear if perhaps desiccated thyroid prevented osteoporosis.

Thyroid hormone action

The principle of specificity in thyroid hormone action at its target site is very important. There are numerous examples of thyroid hormone doing one thing in one animal and the exact same function in another animal is not affected by thyroid hormone. Again, if thyroxine has been directing the genome of the cell since the beginning it is not surprising that there would be different effects in different species and tissues.

Sub-clinical hypothyroidism.

Sub-clinical hypothyroidism has been the subject of much debate. By definition these people have raised or abnormal TSH values but theoretically no symptoms. But if these patients have the symptoms described by the clinicians of the past, such as Crile and Warner illustrated above, surely they would get better if given thyroid in adequate doses. We know that if hypothyroidism is not treated there is a more rapid progression of coronary lesions as measured by coronary angiograms. Studies have shown that although these patients are thought to have no symptoms, in fact if questioned intensively, symptoms are elicited which responded to thyroid therapy. As well, the symptoms did not improve or worsen with use of a placebo in place of thyroid hormone.

Some of the puzzles which face the physician are discrepancies between tests of thyroid function and clinical thyroid status found in a number of patients, the pronounced variation in symptoms and signs resulting from thyroid hormone deficiency and excess, and the syndromes of apparent resistance to thyroid hormones. In our discussion here we have given a rational explanation for these puzzles that may need to be approached in a different manner.

Figure 9A

Diagram of anatomical thyroid- pituitary hypothalamic axis.

Drawing represents the normal way of showing **the relationships**

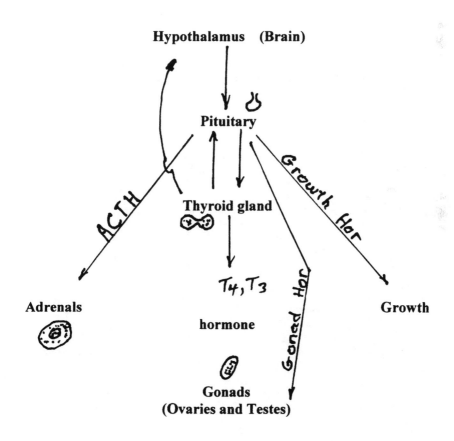

Figure 9B

**Diagram of physiological relationships
action of
Thyroxine, pituitary, thyroid and hypothalamus**

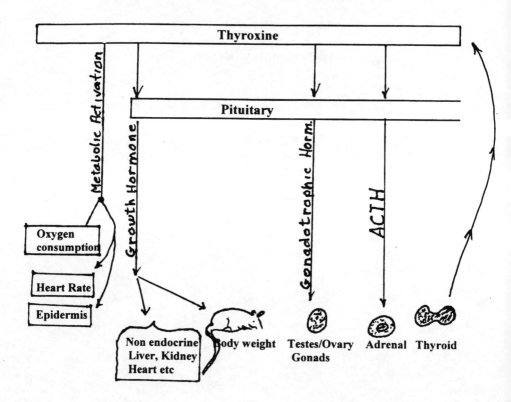

Thyroid gland and thyroid hormone References

1. Wiersinga, W. M. (1985). Nuclear thyroid hormone receptors. Neth.J.Med., 28, 74-82.
2. Chio, A., Magnani, C., & Schiffer, D. (1995). Gompertzian analysis of amyotrophic lateral sclerosis mortality in Italy, 1957-1987; application to birth cohorts. Neuroepidemiology, 14, 269-277.
3. Wooten, W. L. & et al. (1980). The effect of thyroid hormone on mitochondrial biogenesis and cellular hyperplasia. J Bioenerg Biomembr, 12, 1-12.
4. Eartly, H. & Leblond, C. P. (1953). Idendification of the effects of thyroxine mediated by the hypophysis. The New England Journal of Medicine, 249, 249-271.
5. Johnson, L. G. (1997). Thyroxine's evolutionary Roots. Perspectives in Biology & Medicine, 40, 529-535.
6. Samuels, H. H., Tsai, J. S., & Casanova, J. (1974). Thyroid hormone action: in vitro demonstration of putative receptors in isolated nuclei and soluble nuclear extracts. Science, 184, 1188-1191.
7. Di Liegro, I., Savettieri, G., & Cestelli, A. (1987). Cellular mechanism of action of thyroid hormones. Differentiation., 35, 165-175.
8. Crile, G. & and Asscociates (1932). Diagnosis and Treatment of Diseases of the Thyroid Gland. Philadelphia: W.B. Saunders Company.

9. Sawin, C. T. (1991). In C.T.Sawin (Ed.), Clincal Society of London. Report on Myxoedema 1888 Facsimile Edition 1991 (London: Longmans, Green, and Co.

10. Ichikawa, K. & Hashizume, K. (1995). Thyroid hormone action in the cell. [Review] [96 refs]. Endocrine Journal, 1995 Apr;42, 131-140.

11. Segal, J. (1989). Action of the thyroid hormone at the level of the plasma membrane. Endocr.Res., 15, 619-649.

12. Fox, E. L. (1892). A case of myxedema treated by taking extract if thyroid by the mouth. Brit M J, 2, 941.

13. Mackenzie, H. W. (1892). A case of myxoedema treated with great benefit by feeding with fresh thyroid glands. Brit M J, 2, 940.

14. Sawin, C. T. & et al. (1978). A comparison of thyroxine an desiccated thyroid in patients with primary hypothyroidism. Metabolism, 27, 1518-1525.

15. The pharmacological basis of therapeutics (1970). (Fourth edition ed.) Toronto: The MacMillan Company.

16. Selection of thyroid hormone products (1973). Med Lett Drugs Ther, 15, 70-71.

17. Medici, A. (1977). Thyroid replacement therapy. Medical Letter, 19, 50-51.

18. Derry, D. M. (1977). Thyroid replacement therapy. Medical Letter, 19, 50-51.

19. Toft, A. D. (1991). Thyrotropin: Assay, Secretory Physiology, and Testing of Regulation. In L.E.Braverman & R. D. Utiger (Eds.), Werner and Ingbar's The Thyroid (6 ed., pp. 287-305). New York: J.B. Lippincott Company.

20. Werner, A. A. (1942). Endocrinology, clinical application and treatment. Philadelphia: Lea and Febiger.

21. Means, J. H. (1948). The Thyroid and Its Diseases. (2 ed.) Philadelphia, Pa.: J.B. Lippincott.

22. Hoch, F. L. (1962). Biochemical actions of thyroid hormones. Physiol Rev, 42, 605-673.

23. Williams, R. H. & Bakke, J. L. (1962). The Thyroid. In R.H.Williams (Ed.), Textbook of Endocrinology (3 ed., pp. 96-281). Philadelphia: W.B. Saunders Company.

24. Flinn, M. V. & England, B. G. (1997). Social enconomic of childhood glucocorticoid stress response and health. American Jounal of Physical anthropology, 102, 33-53.

25. Rawson, R. W. The thyroid gland. [18], 35-63. 1966. Ref Type: Serial (Book,Monograph)

26. Refetoff, S. (1982). Resistance to thyroid hormone in man. In G.U.Institute of Endocrinology (Ed.), Phylogenetic aspects of thyroid hormone action (pp. 169-189). Tokyo: Center for academic publications Japan.

27. Refetoff, S. (1989). The syndrome of generalized resistance to thyroid hormone (GRTH). Endocr.Res., 15, 717-743.

28. Weiss, R. E. & Refetoff, S. Thyroid hormone resistance. Ann Rev Med 43, 363-375. 1992. Ref Type: Journal (Full)

29. Refetoff, S. (1982). Syndromes of thyroid hormone resistance. Am J Physiol, 243, E88-E98.

30. Franklyn, J. A. (1991). Syndromes of thyroid hormone resistance. Clin Endocrinol.(Oxf.), 34, 237-245.

31. Bauer, M. S., Whybrow, P. C., & Winokur, A. (1990). Rapid cycling bipolar affective disorder. I. Association with grade I hypothyroidism. Arch.Gen.Psychiatry., 47, 427-432.

32. Roti, E., Minelli, R., Gardini, E., & Braverman, L. E. (1993). The use and misuse of thyroid hormone. Endocrine Reviews, 14, 401-423.

33. Oppenheimer, J. H. (1979). Thyroid hormone action at the cellular level. Science, 203, 971-979.

34. Oppenheimer, J. H. (1989). Tissue and Cellular Effects of Thyroid Hormones and Their Mechanism of Action. In G.N.Burrow, J. H. Oppenheimer, & R. Volpe (Eds.), Thyroid Function & Disease (pp. 90-123). Toronto: W.B. Saunders Company.

35. Cooper, D. (1998). Subclinical thyroid disease: a Clinician's perspective. Annals of Internal Medicine, 129, 135-138.

36. Arem, R. & Escalante, D. (1996). Subclinical hypothyroidism. Advances in Internal Medicine, 41, 213-250.

37. Arem, R. & Escalante, D. (1996). Subclinical hypothyroidism: epidemiology, diagnosis, and significance. Advances in Internal Medicine, 1996;41, 213-250.

38. Cooper, D. S., Halpern, R., Wood, L. C., Levin, A. A., & Ridgway, E. C. (1984). L-Thyroxine therapy in subclinical hypothyroidism. A double-blind, placebo-controlled trial. Ann Intern.Med, 101, 18-24.

39. Franklyn, J. A. (1988). The molecular mechanisms of thyroid hormone action. Baillieres.Clin Endocrinol.Metab., 2, 891-909.

Cancer

Genetic changes and cancer

Current research suggests cancer begins in genes. For example, genetic changes are measured in certain cancers, such as colon cancer, at various levels of development of the cancer. However there is a feeling that it will be many years before there will be progress with this approach. The genome is complicated and huge. There are no signs that the majority of chronic diseases such as cancer, arthritis, and autoimmune diseases will be a simple deletion of some sequence within the DNA. In fact the opposite is the case, the cystic fibrosis gene has become progressively more baffling with every new piece of information announced. Even if there was a single deletion from a DNA string, putting it back in correctly still is a daunting task. The work of unraveling the genome may be helpful to the patients of the future, but it is of no use to the person with cancer at present.

Many people have been scared by the thought that cancer generally is genetically based. It is almost as if the cancer was mildly infectious, which so far has not been shown to be true. For some diseases like breast cancer, outcome for a patient can be statistically estimated, especially if they are part of the small percentage having the BRCA genes. But treatment options for these people either before or after they get breast cancer are not good. If present day medicine doesn't have a theory about its cause then there is little hope of finding a cure. Predicting who will get cancer and when is still primitive.

Patients' statistics are almost meaningless. There is no understanding of the reason for cancer or for its progression.

Biological research on cancer

While the advances in deciphering the genome were occurring, many researchers continued investigating cancer in the traditional biological manner. They studied the progression of cancer, its behavior and how it started and what accelerated the process. Enormous amounts of work unraveled development and progress of cancers in animals and humans, thus laying out the sequence of events leading to cancer. This gives us, the following generation, a better chance to try to understand what is happening and why. Without the work of these workers we could not begin to guess its cause. What are the reasons behind the progressive changes seen in the development of an abnormal cell in a continuum towards a cancer cell? Few have dared to guess at the mechanisms behind this process, but it is encouraging news that most cancer systems are similar in their progression of events.

Cancer complexity

Much of the complexity of histological sections of cancer is related to many different cell types from the tissues undergoing the process of conversion from pre-cancerous lesions to cancerous at different rates and different starting times. Any one section of a breast will contain many different cell types in some degree of abnormality, not necessarily cancerous, but likely pre-cancerous. As some of the cells started on the cancer process later than others, there will be many cell types at different stages of development towards cancer. They are all mixed up in the same section of tissue being examined under the microscope. As the cancer tumors progress they coalesce and make one intertwined cancerous lesion. The further along the process, the more difficult it is to differentiate the tumor's origin. The largest lesion is made up of one of the faster growing tumor cells in that tissue. Because of these confusing pictures most pathologists and research workers have postulated that there cannot ever be one cause for breast cancer and it is grandiose to even attempt to put together any unifying theory. However unless someone tries we still have no theory. As Dr. Peter Medewar, a Noble Laureate of the Twentieth Century, has said "Science without the underpinning of hypothesis is just kitchen arts." Even an incorrect theory stimulates new ideas and approaches to scientific problems.

This book is about the cause of cancer and its progression. It has little to do with genetics except in the sense as described earlier that the genome is controlled by thyroid hormone and iodine. The two types of thyroid hormone (T3 and T4) and perhaps also reverse T3 along with iodine make up the total surveillance and protection mechanism against cancer.

Natural history of cancer

After a century of intensive study of cancer we are not much further ahead in treatment. The reason is that we still don't understand it. Most cancers take many years to develop. Even if they are growing at a fast pace at the time of clinical detection they take many years to become clinically significant. The overall estimate is probably around 20-30 years or, said another way, they take up to half the life-span of the animal or human. Ten of those growing and developing years or more may be spent in a pre-cancerous state. All researchers have emphasized the slowness of the pre-cancerous changes. The advantage is that whatever mechanism is involved in surveillance for cancer has ample opportunity to activate the process of anti-cancer and hopefully reversal. Clarke, Sirica, Fisher, Fischer, Faber, Rubin, Haagensen and many others have defined the sequence of events in the progression of cancer. The concepts are relatively simple but there are many variations due to sensitivity in different tissues.

Figure 10

Carcinogenic stimulants

We know that painting animals skin with carcinogens will bring on cancer in many different ways both locally and distally in other organs. The detailed analysis of this phenomenon showed it was similar to other carcinogenic processes. It is clear there are many carcinogens in our environment, many of which have been present since the beginning of time. All stimulate cells over time to become abnormal. If these cancer-causing chemicals have been in our environment since the early stages of evolution, it seems probable there is a built-in system to deal with this problem.

The problems caused by carcinogens were unimportant to single celled organisms such as bacteria because they could adapt in various ways to escape the effects of the chemicals or conditions. In fact they could transfer genes between themselves by means of plasmids (small bits of DNA usually circular that can transfer information) therefore they were able to resist almost any chemical or condition that came into the environment. Much of the population of single cells could be sacrificed in order to adapt and thrive. Once multicellular nucleated organisms arrived they needed a different system to replace most of the actions of the plasmids. Sacrificing large parts of the organism in order to adapt to changes in the environment was not a plausible alternative for multicellular organisms like vertebrates and mammals. It is my intention to simplify these concepts with the aid of diagrams in order to better be able to explain the overall action of iodine and thyroid on these systems.

Figure 11

Most of these imaginary tissue diagrams showing cells turning slowly into cancer are derived from the concepts described in detail by Dr. Clarke. They are my interpretation of his papers.

In the first diagram I have drawn a hypothetical unit or compartment system made up of some of the key players in the problems to do with cancer genesis. Although not strictly transferable this system mimics breast cancer more than other systems. I have purposely left out some features, which only add to the complexity of the concepts, but do not help with understanding.

There is the parenchyma, which is the tissue of that organ. In the breast it would be breast glandular duct system, in the liver, liver cells and so on. Surrounding the tissue are connective tissue elements and fibroblasts, the main cell of connective tissue. Many chemical and biologically active substances are secreted into connective tissue. Some of these are part of the interactive communication system within a unit. Outside the connective tissue there is a basement membrane.

The communications and interactions between the different parts of this unit are mostly near-by acting compounds that are signaling the cell next door or several doors away. The basement membrane seems to be important to the overall coordination of the unit. There is an elaborate continuous interaction between the cells of these units along with the systemic factors like nerves, blood vessels, lymphatic ducts and hormones to tightly run the cells within the unit. Dr. Clarke has gone on to say that when the communication system or interaction breaks down between these cells within a unit, the resulting disorganization allows neoplasia or abnormal growth of cells to occur.

This is a different concept to the normal view of the origin of cancerous cells. In our normal view of cancer we look at cells changing their characteristics from normal to cancerous and then attacking the surrounding tissues. Whereas Dr. Clarke is saying that the changes in the environment of the unit can lead to changes in a cell towards abnormality and neoplasia. At the microscopic level the normal integrity of the connective tissue represents the defensive barrier against the development and spread of cancer.

Dr. Clarke's sequence of events

At first we must pay attention to the parenchyma as this is the real source of most cancerous cells. Dr. Clarke Jr, while at Harvard Medical School, started a 25-year project of photographing every inch of skin of 2534 patients. As he was a skin pathologist, he was able to watch carefully as the skin changed and then to biopsy it and correlate the histological changes with the changes in the photographs. Every patient was followed for 25 years in this manner. He concluded there were certain events in cancer development that have applicability to other cancer systems such as cervical cancer, colon cancer and breast cancer. Many of his findings on skin are similar to cancer development in other systems.

First Stage of cancer development

For the first stages of cancer development there is a precursor state caused by some inductive mechanism, which may be a chemical or a systemic condition. Many inductive chemicals have been present in our environments since the earth's beginnings. This implies vertebrate systems should have a form of defence against abnormal, against the carcinogens or both. However, so many types of chemicals, stimuli and even odd shapes of inert plastic, can induce cancer that there may not be a mechanism for each carcinogen as has been set up against foreign proteins by the immune system. Because of the wide variety of inducers of cancer process and because the overall process seems to be the same for many types of cancer systems it would be easier to eliminate the cells after they have started on the abnormal path. It would also be useful if the same mechanism removing abnormal cells also took up the function of the plasmids in bacteria by neutralizing the inducing chemicals.

Within the process of the precursor state, the number of cells showing signs of change towards abnormal is quite variable and may be related to the severity of the inductor. In some cases there will only be scattered single cells throughout the tissue. In others the lesions of the precursor state can have already progressed to a size that can be seen with the naked eye. These bigger visible lesions are usually composed of arrays of individual cells all of which were abnormal. It is a characteristic of the precursor state that the vast majority of these cells die or the abnormality is repaired by some pre-programmed form of maturation and development back to their normal type of cells.

Dr. Clarke emphasized that at this stage no real signs of cancer developed, only small groups of single abnormal cells, and that almost all of the abnormal cells at this stage either disappeared or went through a programmed differentiation. Rarely, after the passage of much time the occasional cell would not disappear and it would proceed in the direction of cancer. But one of the most important features of the precursor state was that the precursor state marks an entire organ at risk for development of cancer even though progression from this precursor state to cancer is rare. There are so many causes of the precursor state it is unlikely that a defense system could cope directly with all the different causes but it might be able to cope with the tissue response, which is fairly uniform.

Figures 12, 13, 14 cancer development

Second stage carcinoma in situ

The next stage he described was a continuation of the previous precursor state but some or one of the lesions progresses rather than reversing its path and becomes a group of similar atypical cells in one mass. The cells in these little groups often appear almost clonal in nature. This always occurs within one compartment or unit. These are better known as carcinoma in situ - meaning cancer at the site. It appears that this type of lesion is composed of cells that have arisen by mitotic division and are very similar in appearance. But the basement membrane is the defining characteristic of the compartment and carcinoma in situ does not cross this membrane. It stays within the unit. So there is no growth of the cells into another compartment. The new characteristic of this stage is that its growth is slow but it is usually continuous. Some regress back to normal, scarring or differentiate back to normal, but a significant number just slowly keep growing.

Cancer stage

The next stage is cancer. That means there is growth of the cells outside of the compartment. The basement membrane separates most compartments so cancer has crossed a basement membrane into another unit. We now have growth of cells in more than one compartment, which is now by definition cancer. That is cancer is a growth in more than one compartment or unit. Cancerous cells arise from within the previous carcinoma in situ and become more malignant to the point that it starts to multiply and spread via the surrounding connective tissue.

Cancer spread and connective tissue

Because cancer cells have gained access to more than one compartment or unit they are also capable now of entering blood vessels and lymphatics to spread to distant sites. This now is called metastatic disease. But it is important to realize that all of the metastatic lesions that start up in distant sites always start up in the connective tissue of the host tissue. So if a single cell gets into the blood stream and lands in a particular organ, it will not grow unless it arrives in the connective tissue of that organ. This explains some of the cases of local recurrence in breast cancer. The cells may have gone all over the body and ended up with the most friendly and compatible connective tissue environment in which to start up again — the breast itself. Since local recurrences may have started this way, they are looked on as more ominous. It is an indicathat some cells may have gone into blood stream or lymphatics and then gained access to the blood and then re-implanted in the breast tissues again. As connective tissue appears to be the only place metastatic lesions can start, this emphasizes the importance of connective tissue as the major defense in both normal and metastatic disease.

Precursor state causes.

Following from the concepts discussed in the first part, in the breast the precursor state is caused by a relatively low iodine intake. That is a daily value below the level that saturates the thyroid gland. On this continent and Europe the amount of iodine in the diet has never approached levels of dietary intake required to saturate the thyroid. During the normal course of events of consuming a North American diet, most of the iodine in the diet is captured by the still unsaturated thyroid gland. It makes sense that if the thyroid is saturated then almost all dietary iodine will be used to flood the extra-cellular fluids and with time eventually trigger off the death of any abnormal or atypical cells. The details of this action on the breast fibrocystic disease will be described in the section on breast cancer, but suffice it to say that doses of iodine above the saturation level make fibrocystic disease reverse and disappear both in animals and in humans.

Iodine's role in cancer prevention.

Iodine in adequate doses neutralizes carcinogens, removes abnormal cells, kill viruses, which might be carcinogenic, and neutralizes toxins from other micro-organisms. These are the same as many of the functions of plasmids. Adequate amounts of iodine in the circulating blood would likely prevent these serious consequences. We now know iodine in the blood would neutralize toxins and allergic foreign proteins, as it does in the stomach. Most of breast cancer studies on female Japanese immigrants to North America reveal it takes two or three generations of Japanese Americans before their cancer rate is similar to that of the Americans. It is likely that over those generations the incidence of fibrocystic disease would increase and then finally the incidence of breast cancer would settle in at the much higher rate in North America. This is likely related to the drastic lowering of dietary iodine in the descendants of the immigrants.

Biphasic cancer (two phases of development)

Cancer appears to have two phases (biphasic). This idea is not entirely new. Dr. Sampson hinted at it after completion of two comparative studies on the incidence of occult cancer (carcinoma in situ) of the thyroid in Japanese and Minnesotans. He felt cancer might be dissociated into two phases. From all the material of Dr. Clarke, we can divide cancer progression into early lesions and states up to carcinoma in situ as being caused by relative iodine deficiency. The second part, which involves the spread of cancers cells through the connective tissue and including metastatic cancer, are related to low tissue thyroid hormone levels. Anywhere the connective tissue defense is too strong, the cancer cells cannot travel in the connective tissue and will stay within the same compartment and probably die of old age as describe in the breast examined at autopsy in elderly women.

Connective tissue defence against cancer spread.

Since the 1888 report of the committee on Myxedema we know that that one of the classical features of extreme low thyroid conditions is the accumulation of a mucin, then called mucopolysaccarides, in the all body connective tissues. These connective sites include skin, heart, liver, vocal cords and many others. Research on connective tissue reveals that indeed thyroid hormone is the controller of the whole connective tissue system as we would expect from the concepts raised in parts one and two. Hence, the last precancerous lesion in Clarke's model, carcinoma in situ, will spread early if there is also a low thyroid hormone in the tissue. So in spreading breast cancer itself thyroid hormone levels would be especially low in the connective tissue.

The question is, is there any confirmation of the idea that there are two aspects of iodine and thyroid control of cancer? That thyroid is in overall control of connective tissue has been shown by many studies. Not only does connective tissue give cohesion, strength and form to organs that it surrounds, but it also serves as a barrier when it is strong and as a pathway for the spread of cancer when it is weak. From all the published literature on connective tissue, thyroid hormone is the controlling and permissive hormone of connective tissue. From our thesis stated above, this would be a reasonable role for it to play. It is interesting that 50 years ago Professor Hadfield said: "It is my firm belief that for many years we have been so anxious to discover all we possibly can about the structure of the growth and its metastases that we have almost forgotten the soil in which it grows"

There are several expressions of thyroid disease which show themselves in connective tissue, including myxedema, one of the original findings. It may not be appreciated that local areas of the body can have a low tissue thyroid hormone level. For example; pretibial dermopathy, which is a swelling of the front of the leg, seen in certain thyroid diseases confirms that this can occur. Detailed studies of the effects of injections of T3 into these tissues tell us there is a local insensitivity to thyroid hormone existing for unknown reasons. In addition work in the 1930s revealed that thyroid therapy could be used to avoid keloid formation in post surgical incisions. These results suggest a localized (within the dermis) insensitivity to thyroid hormone or a localized lower level of tissue thyroid hormone. It was noted at the time that Japanese surgeons were not even aware of keloid formation in their country. So localized areas of thyroid hormone effectiveness or levels present are possible in some conditions in what are apparently normal people. Fortunately, this is correctable by orally given thyroid hormone.

Sampson's on carcinoma in situ in Japanese thyroids

Looking at the work of Sampson, he personally did identical pathological studies on the thyroids of normal Japanese and Minnesotans. He was amazed in the beginning to find that the Japanese had a 34% rate of carcinoma in situ. None of the Japanese patients were in any way involved or near the atomic bomb explosions. He went back and checked it again and used as standardized conditions and stains as he could arrange. He then went to the County around the Mayo Clinic and examined the thyroids in the identical fashion. He found again that the Minnesotans had about 4% or less incidence of carcinoma in situ in thyroid cancer. What bothered Sampson was that the Japanese have the lowest rate of mortality from or even clinical evidence of thyroid cancer in the world. In fact, that Minnesotans clinical cancer rate was higher. This did not make sense unless there were two phases to cancer. He felt that there might be two dissociable phases to cancer. From the evidence presented above one phase could be as far as carcinoma in situ and the other phase went beyond that. Obviously, the first phase affects the Japanese thyroid gland, but not the second thyroid hormone phase.

At the same time we know that the Japanese intake of iodine is as high as anywhere in the world. The average intake is about 8-10 mgs. This is well above the thyroid saturation point of 2-3 mgs. That means that the Japanese have lots of excess iodine bathing their bodies daily and being excreted in their urine. In fact, Japanese urinary excretion rates of iodine are about the highest in the world. How do we explain this in terms of the concepts put forward here? Because if there was a high level of circulating iodine in Japanese, why have these molecules of iodine not eliminated all the carcinoma in situ in Japanese thyroid glands as described in the main thesis of this book?

Transport system of iodine and salt

The transport system for iodine across membranes into cells seems to have been well preserved through evolution and is related to the original seaweed mechanism. The transport system of iodine into the thyroid is a modification of that system. Iodine uptake into the thyroid gland is blocked by a number of compounds. One important chemical example is nitrate. Nitrate, which is increasingly found in fertilizers, which then end up in drinking water, fodder, vegetables and vegetable juices to say nothing of its use in food preservatives. The main source of nitrates in the Japanese diet is food preservatives.

The transport system for iodide into thyroid cells is carried out by a sodium-iodide symporter. This symporter transports two different ions, sodium and iodide in the same direction across the plasma membrane of thyroid cells. Apparently, the same system transports iodide in normal lactating breast ducts, the stomach and in parotid glands. Both nitrate and salt have been implicated as causes of gastric cancer. In this scheme of transport of iodide in the system it is easier to see how both nitrate blocking iodide uptake and sodium saturating the system may both be inhibitors of iodide excretion into the stomach or iodide uptake into thyroid tissue and may be related to stomach cancer.

Nitrates relation to stomach cancer

Let us leave the Japanese thyroid problem of carcinoma in situ for a minute and discuss the problem of the relationship of nitrates to gastric cancer. The transport system of iodine into the stomach is the same as the salivary gland, breast and prostate. If iodine transport into the stomach lumen is blocked by nitrates, then there would be a relative lack of iodine in the lumen of the stomach. This means at least two things. One is that the helicobacter pylori bacterium would not be killed as easily and also the iodine would not be there to promote the apoptosis or natural cell death turnover of the gastric cells. At a turnover rate of 2-3 days it could be noticeable. Now what about the second phase of our biphasic cancer system in the stomach?

In the lumen of the stomach there is no connective tissue or thyroid hormone to promote a defense against cancer overgrowth or atypical cells developing into cancer tumors. In the lumen of the stomach the role of the iodine is more important because of this lack of connective tissue barrier run by thyroid hormone to prevent the growth of cancers. The Japanese have one of the highest consumptions of nitrates in the world and the highest rate of gastric cancer. Many studies have shown a correlation between the two.

Current theories of gastric cancer

The general theory proposed for gastric cancer is that the induction of gastric cancers by nitrates is related to the conversion of the nitrates into carcinogenic compounds substances called nitrosamines. But it has been hard to confirm conclusively that the formation of nitrosamines actually occurs in meaningful amounts. So the theory of the nitrate connection to stomach cancer has been changed several times. But work in Chile whose soil contains rich amounts of nitrates, shows the same correlations of nitrates to gastric cancer. Also the gastric cancer rate in Chile is almost the same as the Japanese and both have had conferences to show that their problem is related to the nitrates. The concentration of nitrosamines in foods is usually small, and it remains to be established whether their presence is a significant risk to human populations.

Dr. Sampson's findings

So now we can go back to the problem of Dr. Sampson and his carcinoma in situ in the thyroids of normal Japanese. From what we have discussed above, the iodine intake will be inhibited in the thyroids of the adult Japanese from their consumption of nitrate treated foods. At the same time, most of Japanese do not take up the dietary habit of consuming preserved foods until adulthood. Therefore, a large part of their thyroids will be working at top efficiency for all their adult lives. The consumption of nitrate in adult life may selectively affect only some of the cells of the thyroid gland and thus lead to an intracellular iodine deficiency. It is also possible nitrate blocks the apoptotic trigger mechanism. Both of these would allow cells to develop abnormally.

So we would expect to see a high rate of carcinoma in situ or occult carcinomas in tissues which have iodine transport systems. The incidence of carcinoma in situ in the breasts of Japanese women is high and the incidence of cancer is low. The same applies to the prostate in which there is a high level of carinoma in situ but carcinoma of the prostate in Japanese is like Japanese breast cancer, about the lowest in the world. The explanation for this appears to be that the Japanese continue to have well functioning thyroid glands in spite of the nitrates. This maintains the integrity and defensive power of the connective tissues and does not let the multiple carcinomas in situ spread in any form. But because of the nitrate blocking iodine transport across the membrane, it will allow growth due to local microscopic iodine deficiency up to occult cancer or carcinoma in situ.

Figure 10

Changes in Cells from normal to Cancerous

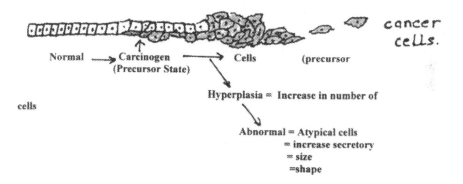

More iodine   less iodine

Iodine in diet makes go towards normal.

Lack of iodine allows cells to go towards atypical and cancer.

Figure 11

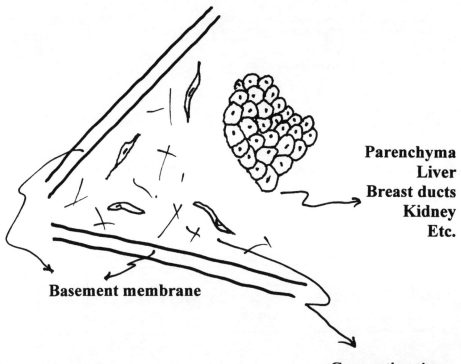

Compartment (unit)

Simplified from Clarke

Parenchyma
Liver
Breast ducts
Kidney
Etc.

Basement membrane

Connective tissue
And fibroblasts.

Figure 12

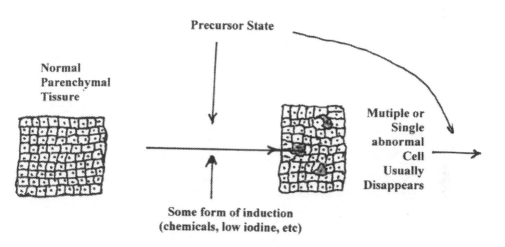

Description of progression to cancer
from Clarke's description
(my interpretation)

Figure 13

**Clarke's Progression to cancer from
normal cells.**

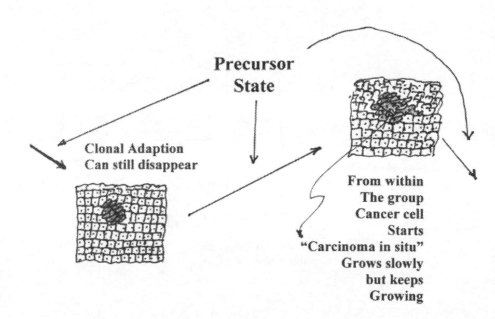

**Precursor
State**

Clonal Adaption
Can still disappear

From within
The group
Cancer cell
Starts
"Carcinoma in situ"
Grows slowly
but keeps
Growing

Figure 14

Clarke's Progression to cancer from normal cells.

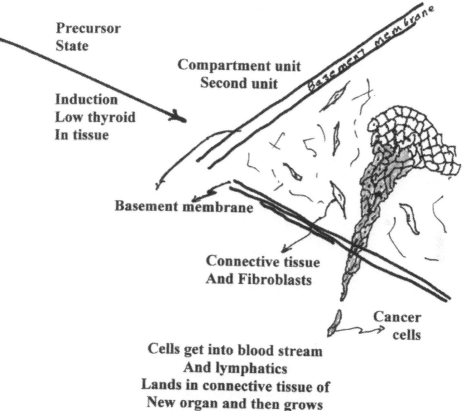

Precursor
State

Compartment unit
Second unit

Induction
Low thyroid
In tissue

Basement membrane

Connective tissue
And Fibroblasts

Cancer
cells

Cells get into blood stream
And lymphatics
Lands in connective tissue of
New organ and then grows

Cancer References

1. Cavenee, W. K. & White, R. L. The genetic basis of cancer. Scientific American 272, 72-79. 1995.
2. Nicolson, G. L. (1987). Tumor cell instability, diversification, and progression to the metastatic phenotype: from oncogene to oncofetal expression. Cancer Res, 47, 1473-1487.
3. Weinberg, R. A. (1995). Prospects for cancer genetics. Cancer Surv., 25, 3-12.
4. Fearon, E. R. (1992). Genetic alterations underlying colorectal tumorigenesis. Cancer Surv., 12, 119-136.
5. Vogelstein, B. & Kinzler, K. W. (1994). Colonrectal cancer and the intersection between basic and clinical research. Cold Spring Harbor Symp Quant Biol, 59, 517-521.
6. Fearon, E. R. (1990). A genetic model for colonorectal tumorigenesis. Cell, 61, 759.
7. Lyons, A. S. & Petrucelli, R. J. (1987). Medicine an Illustraed History. New York: Abradale Press Harry N. Abrams, Inc., Publishers.
8. Clark, W. H. (1995). The nature of cancer: morphogenesis and progressive (self) disorganization in neoplastic developmement and progression. Acta Oncol., 34, 3-21.
9. Clark, W. H. (1991). Tumour progression and the nature of cancer. In (64 ed., pp. 631-644).
10. Sirica, A. E. (1988). The pathbiology of neoplasia. New York: Plenum Press.

11. Foulds, L. (1969). Neoplastic development. New York: Academic Press.

12. Fisher, B. The surgical dilemna in primary therapy of invasive breast cancer: a critical appraisal. Ravitch, M. M., Julian, O. C., Scott, H. W., Thal, A. R., and Wangensteen, O. H. 4-52. 1970. Chicago, Year Book Medical Publishers. Montly Clinical Monographs.

13. Fisher, B. & Fisher, E. Transmigration of lymph nodes by tumor cells. Science 352, 1397. 1966.

14. Farber, E. & Rubin, H. (1991). Cellular adaptation in the origin and development of cancer. Cancer Res, 51, 2751-2761.

15. Farber, E. & Sarma, D. S. (1987). Biology of disease: hepatocarinogenesis: a dynamic cellular perspective. Lab Invest, 56, 4.

16. Rubin, H. (1990). On the nature of enduring modifications induded in cells and organisms. Am J Phyiol, 258, 19.

17. Fong, C. J., Sherwood, E. R., Braun, E. J., Berg, L. A., Chung, L., & Kozlowski, J. M. (1992). Regulation of prostatic carcinoma cell proliferation and secretory activity by extracellular matrix and stromal secrections. Prostate, 21, 121-131.

18. Chung, L. W. (1993). Implications of stromal epithelial interaction in human prostate cancer growth, progression and differentiation. Semin Cancer Biol, 4, 183-192.

19. Atkins, P. W. (1995). The periodic kingdom. New York: Basic Books A Division of Harper Collins Publishers.

20. Chung, L. W., Gleave, M. E., Hsieh, J., Hong, S. J., & Shau, H. E. (1991). Reciprical mesenchymal-epithelial interaction affecting prostate tumor growth and hormonal responsiveness. Cancer Surv., 11, 91-121.

21. Summers, D. K. (1996). The biology of plasmids. Oxford: Blackwell Science Ltd.

22. Benazzi, C., Sarli, G., Galeotti, M., & Marcato, P. S. (1993). Basement membrane components in mammary tumours of the dog and cat. J Comp Pathol, 109, 241-252.

23. Forsyth, I. A. (1991). The mammary gland. Baillieres Clinical Endocrinology & Metabolism, 5, 809-832.

24. Gonzalez-Sancho, J. M., Alvarez-Dolado, M., Caelles, C., & Munoz, A. (1999). Inhibition of tenascin-C expression in mammary epithelial cells by thyroid hormone. Molecular Carcinogenesis, 24, 99-107.

25. Bayraktar, M., Gedik, O., Akalin, S., Usman, A., Adalar, N., & Telatar, F. (1990). The effect of radioactive iodine treatment on thyroid C cells. Clin Endocrinol.(Oxf.), 33, 625-630.

26. Davenport, H. W. & Fisher, R. B. Mechanisms of the secretion of acid by the gastric mucosa. Am J Physiol 131, 165-175. 1940.

27. Sporn, M. B. (1991). Carcinogenesis and cancer: different perspectives on the same disease. Cancer Res, 51, 6215-6218.

28. Sawin, C. T. (1991). In C.T.Sawin (Ed.), Clincal Society of London. Report on Myxoedema 1888 Facsimile Edition 1991 (London: Longmans, Green, and Co.

29. Bissel, M. J., Hall, H. G., & Parry, G. (1982). How does the extracellular matrix direct gene expression? J Theor Biol, 99, 31-68.

30. Bartow, S. A., Pathak, D. R., Black, W. C., Key, C. R., & Teaf, S. R. Prevalence of benign, atypical and malignant breast lesions in populations at different risk for breast cancer. Cancer 60, 2751-2760. 1987.

31. Smith, T. J., Bahn, R. S., & Gorman, C. A. (1989). Connective tissue, glycosaminoglycans, and diseases of the thyroid. Endocr.Rev., 10, 366-391.

32. Benvenga, S. & Robbins, J. Enhancement of thyroxine entry into low density lipoprotein (LDL) receptor-competence fibroblasts by LDL: an additional mode of entry of thyroxine into the cells. Endocrinology 331, 847-941. 2001.

33. Sampson, R. J., Key, C. R., Buncher, C. R., & Iijima, S. Thyroid carcinoma in Hiroshima and Nagasaki—I. Prevalence of thyroid carcinoma at autopsy. JAMA 209, 65-70. 1969.

34. Sampson, R. J. & et al. (1974). Occult thyroid carcinoma in Olmsted County, Minnesota: prevalence at autopsy compared with that in Hiroshima and Nagasaki, Japan. Cancer, 34, 2072-2076.

35. Fukunaga, F. H. & et al. (1975). Geographic pathology of occult thyroid carcinomas. Cancer, 36, 1095-1099.

36. Guiloff, R. J. & Goonetilleke, A. (1995). Natural history of amyotrophic lateral sclerosis. Observations with the Charing Cross Amyotrophic Lateral Sclerosis Rating Scales. Advances in Neurology, 68, 185-198.

37. Welcsh, P. L. & Mankoff, D. A. (2000). Taking up iodide in breast tissue. Nature, 406, 688-689.

38. Yamagata, H., Kiyohara, Y., Aoyagi, K., Kato, I., & Iwamto, H. e. al. (200). Impact of Heliobacter pylori infection on gastric cancer incidence in a general Japanese population: The Hisayama study. Arch Intern Med, 10, 1962-1968.

39. Vyth, A., Timmer, J. G., Bossuyt, P. M., Louwerse, E. S., & de, J. (1996). Survival in patients with amyotrophic lateral sclerosis, treated with an array of antioxidants. Journal of the Neurological Sciences, 139 Suppl, 99-103.

40. Chio, A., Magnani, C., & Schiffer, D. (1995). Gompertzian analysis of amyotrophic lateral sclerosis mortality in Italy, 1957-1987; application to birth cohorts. Neuroepidemiology, 14, 269-277.

41. Mueller, C. B. & Jeffries, W. Cancer of the breast: Its outcome as measured by the rate of dying and causes of death. Ann Surg 182, 334-341. 1975.

42. Dungal, N. The special problem of stomach cancer in Iceland. JAMA 178, 789-798. 1961.

43. Appel, S. H., Smith, R. G., Alexianu, M., Siklos, L., Engelhardt, J., Colom, L. V., & Stefani, E. (1995). Increased intracellular calcium triggered by immune mechanisms in amyotrophic lateral sclerosis. Clinical Neuroscience, 3, 368-374.

44. Julien, J. P. (1995). A role for neurofilaments in the pathogenesis of amyotrophic lateral sclerosis. Biochemistry & Cell Biology, 73, 593-597.

45. Salazar-Grueso, E. F. & Roos, R. P. (1995). Amyotrophic lateral sclerosis and viruses. Clinical Neuroscience, 3, 360-367.

46. You, W. C., Blot, W. J., Chang, Y. S., & et al (1992). Comparison of the anatomic distribution of stomach cancer and precancerous gastric lesions. Jpn J Cancer Res, 83, 1150-1153.

47. Steingrimsdottir, L. (1993). Nutrition in Iceland. Scand J Nutrr, 37, 10-12.

48. Steingrimsdottir, L., Sigurdsson, G. Jr., & Sigurdsson, G. Nutrition and serum lipids in Iceland. Scand J Nutrr 39, 138-141. 1995.

49. Venturi, S., Venturi, A., Cimini, D., Arduini, C., Venturi, M., & Guidi, A. (1993). A new hypothesis: iodine and gastric cancer. European Joural of Cancer Prevention, 2, 17-23.

50. Jahreis, G., Schone, F., Ludke, H., & Hesse, V. (1987). Growth impairment caused by dietary nitrate intake regulated via hypothyroidism and decreased somatomedin. Endocrinologia Experimentalis, 21, 171-180.

51. Sobue, I., Saito, N., Iida, M., & Ando, K. (1978). Juvenile type of distal and segmental muscular atrophy of upper extremities. Annals of Neurology, 3, 429-432.

52. Adami, H. O. (1984). Breast cancer incidence and mortality. Aspects on aetiology, time trends and curability. Acta Chirurgica Scandinavica - Supplementum, 519, 9-14.

53. Akiyama, F., Iwase, T., Yoshimoto, M., Kasumi, F., & Sakamoto, G. (1995). Incidence of latent breast cancer in Japanese women. Journal of Cancer Research & Clinical Oncology, 1995;121, 564-566.

54. Mason, R. & Wilkinson, J. S. (1973). The thyroid gland— a review. [Review] [52 refs]. Australian Veterinary Journal, 49, 44-49.

55. Morimoto, T., Sasa, M., Yamaguchi, T., Harada, K., & Sagara, Y. (1994). High detection rate of breast cancer by mass screening using mammography in Japan. Japanese Journal of Cancer Research, 1994 Dec;85, 1193-1195.

56. Gourie-Devi, M., Suresh, T. G., & Shankar, S. K. (1984).
     Monomelic amyotrophy. <u>Archives of Neurology, 41,</u> 388-
     394.

Breast Cancer

To date we have not been able to guess the cause of breast cancer. The breasts are one of the most hormonally dependent tissues along with the endometrium of the uterus and the prostate in men. Breast feeding of off-spring gave mammals an advantage, as breast milk feeding became exactly catered to maximal growth and development, especially of the human brain.

Normal changes in the Breast

There are marked microscopic changes in breast structure occurring during a normal menstrual cycle. There is an increase in the number cells, an enlargement of some cells and a change in secretory function in others, all, in preparation for a potential pregnancy. During pregnancy much higher circulating levels of hormones exaggerate the physical changes. At the end of a menstrual cycle the cellular changes must return to the normal resting state by a natural death of many cells. Unfortunately this process in many women is incomplete. As a result the breast gradually builds up layers of cells after each menstrual cycle, which did not die correctly. The lumpy result of this accumulation is fibrocystic disease of the breast.

Fibrocystic disease is a catch-all term for nodules, cysts and scars in sometimes painful breasts. The name fibrocystic disease has stuck because it is most useful clinically. The patient can relate to an explanation that her breast lumps are benign in nature. So the real clinical utility of the name is in conversing with the patient and that is extremely important— in this world of breast cancer fear. Some physicians make light of these changes because they feel the changes will not lead to breast cancer. However, since there is now a way to dissolve the fibrocystic disease by increasing iodine intake, reduction of the incidence of breast cancer to Japanese rates could follow.

Many sites of breast lumps and tenderness move around the breast in different menstrual cycles. Therefore, a biopsy will not necessarily look the same even one month later. On the other hand some fibrocystic lesions seem to be fairly permanent caused by leaking irritating cyst fluid. The heterogeneity of fibrocystic disease comes from the many cell types responding to hormones differently and resolving the menstrual cycle build-up in a different manner. Some cells, for example, increase in size and return to normal by shrinking. Other cells acquire secretory organelles within the cells, which also are easy to resolve back to normal. But when there is multiplication of the number of cells then a programmed death or apoptosis must take place in order for the organ to return to its normal or resting state.

Figure 15 Overall thesis.

The inducer of Dr. Clarke's breast precursor state, as defined by Dr. Ghent, is iodine deficiency. But heterogeneity of fibrocystic disease has made evaluation of its relationship to cancer difficult. Just as Dr. Clarke stated a precursor state makes the organ at risk for cancer, so pathologists agree fibrocystic disease has real cancer potential. Microscopic characteristics can define fibrocystic disease's ability to evolve into cancer based on whether the cells are proliferative (increase in number of cells) or non-proliferative.

So, the lady sitting in front of you with clinically abnormal breasts cannot be reassured unless she has a biopsy. Now, if 55% of North American and European women have palpable clinically detectable fibrocystic disease and another 40% have microscopic but clinically undetectable fibrocystic disease, it is hard to establish anything meaningful for the patient because without a biopsy it is guess work. As well, variability in breasts are exaggerated by time of exposure to the inducer and hormones If a biopsy shows benign fibrocystic disease there is still nothing to say that a cancerous lesion, or another type fibrocystic lesion could be in the other breast or another part of the same breast. So, even the information derived from a biopsy may not have predictive value except statistically. Reassuring as this may be, when the biopsy shows a relatively more malignant form of fibrocystic disease such as atypical hyperplasia, we do not have an effective prevention or treatment program, except iodine supplementation suggested here.

Odds of cancer from fibrocystic disease

Because the incidence of breast cancer is not close to incidence of fibrocystic disease much fibrocystic disease comes to nothing. But this is not cause for complacency. The fibrocystic disease is a precursor state, which places the affected breasts at risk for cancer by Dr. Clarke's definition. As well, what is benign about fibrocystic disease, when the odds of getting breast cancer are now down to 1 in 9? No matter who's breasts the physician examines chances are becoming higher a cancer may grow there in the future. Reassurance, under these circumstances, that fibrocystic disease is benign has no meaning to women if the overall incidence remains so high.

Eskin and associates demonstrated that iodine deficiency causes fibrocystic disease in rats and mice. Follow-up therapeutic trials of iodine therapy on women with extensive fibrocystic disease by Ghent and Eskin were remarkably effective no matter what form of iodine was used. Little meaningful follow up has occurred in the literature since, but overall findings showed a high proportion of North American women resolve their fibrocystic disease problems by raising their iodine intake above the 3 mg per day. This level of iodine we know saturates the thyroid gland system within a couple of weeks so that all dietary iodine would be going to non thyroid gland sites, such as extra-cellular fluids bathing all body cells.

Japanese consume 8-10 mg per day of iodine in a natural form of seaweed and fish which compares with Ghent and Eskin's effective dose of 10 mgs per day. Therefore. Ghent and Eskin called fibrocystic disease an iodine deficiency disease. The dose above 3 mgs per day saturates thyroid tissue within two weeks and then all of the dietary intake of iodine given to these women is available for iodine's other functions. This clinically reliable disappearance of fibrocystic disease with iodine therapy is related to iodine triggered apoptosis. We discussed that long term iodine deficiency leads to progressively more malignant thyroid cancers depending on the degree of iodine deficiency. In the same manner breast tissue would be at greater risk of more ominous malignancy by prolonged iodine deficiency.

Iodine and fibrocystic disease

After reading of the clinical effects of iodine on fibrocystic disease in 1993, I searched for the most effective iodine preparation for dissolving fibrocystic disease. All forms of iodine worked. Dosage was a more important factor. If the daily dose of iodine was not over the thyroid gland saturation point of 2-3 mg iodine per day there was no improvement. The thyroid gland was still capturing iodine out of the blood system at too high a rate to allow the proper circulation of iodine throughout the body.

As we have postulated in the section on iodine, the first part of the biphasic cancer surveillance system of the body is the presence of iodine in the extra-cellular spaces. Our dietary intakes in North America and Europe are about 1/10th the intake needed to saturate the thyroid and fulfill the needs of the surveillance system for abnormal cells. As the World Health Organization recommended dose of iodine is designed to prevent goiter formation, we now think this a sub-optimal intake for longevity, good health and cancer prevention.

Iodine therapy to carcinoma in situ?

Microscopic fibrocystic disease is a continuum from the normal cell, to the abnormal cells, through to atypical cells and cancer cells. The abnormal cells can multiply at any stage forming a clump, which is not cancerous. This is carcinoma in situ. This is the stage of slow but usually progressive growth. Carcinoma in situ also has greater potential to convert to cancer cells than any of the other fibrocystic forms. The rates of conversion vary with the cell type. But now we can suggest that all of the stages of development up to and including carcinoma in situ are reversible with adequate iodine therapy.

Benefits to higher doses of iodine

If ninety percent of the population have fibrocystic disease then why is cancer of the breast not more common? Dr. Clarke stated the number of conversions over to a more cancerous tissue takes many years to accomplish and is rare. Only a very small proportion of the women with fibrocystic disease seem to go on to develop cancer. But this small proportion likely makes up the majority of breast cancer patients who have no risk factors. However we will see that risk factors can be related to iodine intake.

We already learned that the induction of thyroid cancer by relatively low iodine intake takes decades to reverse or cure. Slowly the increase in iodine in the diets of countries using iodine have changed the type and degree of malignancy in thyroid glands from the more malignant follicular to the less malignant papillary cancer. I believe that if the iodine intake of the nations were raised to levels above the saturation point of the thyroid, then there would be a precipitous drop in the cancer rate of the nation to levels similar to those of Japan. And providing the North Americans did not take up the habit of eating nitrate treated foods there would no an increase in the stomach cancer rate either. In a similar manner that thyroid malignancy can take decades to change, resolution of fibrocystic disease in the more difficult cases of the fibrocystic disease can take as long as a couple of years.

The incidence of breast cancer is rising and has been since the early 50s. It has often been quoted that when the salt was iodized in the 1920s that almost completely eliminated goiter and certainly eliminated cretins. The incidence of breast cancer did not change or in fact got worse. This phenomena of using the minimum iodine intake as the standard, made the dietary intake well below thyroid saturation levels and made it ineffective for the prevention of either fibrocystic disease or breast cancer.

Salt intake of women since the 1950

The main source of dietary iodine is iodized salt. Fish is helpful but sometime it is not appreciated how little iodine there is in fish. In order to consume enough fish to cover the amount eaten by the Japanese (8-10 mgs per day) it is estimated that about 10-20 pounds of fish per day would be needed depending on the type of fish. In the Japanese diet seaweed is by far the main source of iodine. The health conscious women of the present era have been brought up since the1950s to take less salt in their diets. This often was emphasized during pregnancy in order to avoid eclampsia and hypertension. So many women eliminated salt from their diets. So their chances of getting enough iodine in their diets to reach levels discussed here are impossible without supplementation. These levels 5-10 mg of iodine daily can be easily reached with Lugol's solution, one drop per day. In the earlier literature it has been published that iodine in the form of Lugol's solution prevented hypertension and eclampsia in pregnancy but this doesn't seem to have been followed up.

The mortality rate from breast cancer has hardly budged in the 80 years since records were kept. Our difficulties seem to be related to not understanding the processes that are going on. This is not surprising when there is such a mixed up confluence of pathological processes all going towards abnormal at different rates. In one person, one type will go forward and in another type other lesions will appear. Obviously if the thyroid hormone level is low in the tissue, then the prognosis will be poorer. As the microscopic degree of aggressiveness may be partly related to the level of thyroid hormone, since one of thyroid hormone's main functions is to mature (differentiate) cells toward normal.

My experiences with breast cancer.

At present my experience, of putting patients with breast cancer on iodine and thyroid hormone at levels to make them feel good and cope well has been gratifying. The recent finding that estrogen hormones decreases the mortality and increases the survival rate of breast cancer patients has confirmed my own impression that estrogens also contribute to a women's constitution and overall resistance. The well being and constitution of the patient are almost synonymous. Thyroid hormone is the most important hormone for maintaining the well-being, coping ability and overall health. No other medicine comes close. As the old-fashion manner of measuring the effectiveness of thyroid hormone was in assessing the well being of the patient, I make it obligatory that the breast cancer patient take enough thyroid medication to make them at least feel good within themselves. If the patients feel good enough and are "coping" in a normal and healthy manner the tissue levels of thyroid hormone seem to be adequate to maintain the patient in good health, good spirits with plenty of opportunity to carry on with their lives. In these women, they slowly begin to treat the disease as a frightening experience of the past with no further consequences.

Case #1 Psychological benefits.

The opportunity in practice to rid fibrocystic disease from patient's breasts has been gratifying. In many patients the disappearance of their lumps removes a huge burden of anxiety from their minds. One lady who had been particularly compulsive about examining herself once per month on a certain day in the shower knew that her breasts contained many fibrocystic cysts of all sizes up to about 1 cm. She religiously came in for a annual physical examination and we discussed the problem a number of times. When in 1993 she was put on the iodine within several months all of her lumps disappeared. So when she came in a year later I agreed that all evidence of the fibrocystic disease had disappeared. She also mentioned that because her breasts were normal she had forgotten to examine them for several months as there was nothing to find. The benefit to this lady's psyche is immeasurable.

Case #2 'What of atypical hyperplasia and iodine"

Another lady had a diagnosis of breast cancer by mammogram in her left upper breast. I had never examined her breasts prior to the diagnosis being picked up. On examination this lady had quite firm breasts from fibrocystic disease. There was no way to feel the tumor because of the fibrocystic disease. She was put on iodine and her thyroid intake raised. By the time of surgery two months later, the firm lumpiness in the breast rapidly melted away. The cancer was easier to discern. The surgical specimen showed that the disease process in her surrounding breast was atypical hyperplasia, or the worst form of fibrocystic disease with the highest change-over rate to cancer. So, iodine therapy is clinically effective against the most dangerous type of fibrocystic disease. It is my impression that iodine is effective against all lesions up to carcinoma in situ. which are the limits of the first phase of cancer.

Case #3 Carinoma in situ and other pathology around tumor.

Another new patient came to me after a lumpectomy only and no lymph node dissection. Not only was there a ductal carcinoma with multiple foci up to 5 cms from the main lesion, but tissues surrounding her cancer contained many abnormal breast changes including carcinoma in situ. The margins of the cancer came within 0.5 mm of the resection margin. Under the advice of the cancer clinic and because both the margin of clear breast was small and the tissue surrounding the tumor contained many obvious abnormalities , the surgeon carried out a wider resection of the same area and excised the sentinal axillary node six months after I met her. During the interim the lady had been on Lugol's iodine two drops daily and 180 mgs of desiccated thyroid. When a wider resection was carried out all resected breast tissue was completely clear of all fibrocystic disease, pre-cancerous and cancer lesions. The lymph node was negative. This lady had been on her iodine for close to six months at that time as well as thyroid hormone. Theoretically, we should have seen some pathology in her newly resected breast tissue. These results are suggestive that carcinoma in situ and abnormal cells may all disappear with adequate iodine and thyroid therapy.

Case #4 Breast cancer stuck to the skin.

A lady came to see me after she had finished with chemotherapy and radiation for carcinoma of the rectum. She was advised but refused to have surgery. In the light of her history she was started on iodine and thyroid hormone. Approximately a year later she turned up a cancer of the breast in the form of about the size of a nickel, which was firmly stuck to the overlying skin. It was located about one in inch from the nipple. It was partly fixed to the underlying chest wall. She had a biopsy done and it turned out to be carcinoma. She refused surgery and asked me if there was anything else we could do. Several months later I suggested we put a line of Lugol's solution between the nipple and the tumor so that the iodine would be absorbed into the skin and would flow past via the lymphatics through and around the tumor.

About 15% of topical iodine evaporates unless it is covered. She was advised to paint the line once per day and return in two months. When she returned the tumor had disintegrated into about 8 small pieces none of which were now attached to the skin. We enlarged the area of paint to a pie shaped over the tumor. The tumor then did nothing much for the next three years except to scar at the sight of the biggest piece causing a dimple in the breast. There has been no sign of recurrence or extension of the tumor. The lady is alive and well today. It seems breast tumors are also susceptible to iodine in higher concentrations. There may be some way this finding could be exploited.

Risk factors

The question of iodine being captured by fat in the diet has been mentioned in the section on iodine. High fat diets remove iodine from the diet. Iodine depletion by fat can be overcome by either taking less fat or increasing the daily iodine intake to over 2-3 mgs per day. Prostate cancer has also shown similar migration changes and fat intake relationships to breast cancer.

Family history of breast cancer to risk

Another important, but not understood factor in the development of breast cancer, is family relationships. Mother and daughter, sisters and other close relations have a predictably higher rate of cancer. In the light of what we know now it is likely related to passing down the traditions of dietary intake of iodine. Regardless of the food type, the average family likely doesn't vary its iodine intake by much from week to week or even year to year. These habits are learned and become part of life experience. Your likes and dislikes are established early for the majority of the foods that you eat. Mother's food was the greatest, so I want to have food like that. As the dietary intakes of the average North American rarely consistently get up to 2-3 mg in order to saturate the thyroid gland, it is likely that all North Americans are at high risk of breast cancer because of this. The lowering of the salt consumption for health reasons related to blood pressure has only added to the problem and likely increased the incidence and risk. To add to this concept, foster children of parents who die of cancer have a 5 times increased risk of getting cancer. Surely this must be a dietary factor.

Reproductive factors and breast cancer risk

Certain reproductive factors influence the risk of getting breast cancer. If a women has an early onset of her periods (menarche), then it is natural that there will be more hormonal cycles changing the architecture of the breast in a cyclic manner that can only be resolved with adequate intake of iodine. The more cycles the more fibrocystic disease and thus the stimulation by cycles to make more breast cancer. The same applies to a late menopause. More cycles of hormonal stimulation. None of this is a worry if there has been an adequate (thyroid saturating) intake of iodine.

Miscarriage or abortion has been sited as increasing the risk of breast cancer. A pregnancy is partly a huge influx of hormones with many proliferative and structural changes in the breasts, so resolution will involve death of many cells by apoptosis. Higher iodine intake to thyroid saturating levels would likely remove this as a risk factor.

Thus, a miscarriage or abortion would be equivalent to many menstrual cycles stimulating the breast cells. If the women has a miscarriage or an abortion then it is important for her to be consuming adequate iodine to resolve all of the changes that have occurred.

At the other end, the pregnancy goes to term in preparation for lactation and during lactation, we know much more iodine gets into the breast. The breast cancer risk disappears. The reason being that the breast has a built in mechanisms of transport similar to every where else so the breast can concentrate iodine up to 30 times in breast milk.

The Japanese have consumed large amounts of different types of seaweed by incorporating it into their diet and cooking for many centuries. The traditional folklore is that it prevents cancer. In fact Teats in 1980s published a nice summary of the arguments why seaweed might prevent breast cancer. Iodine is the active ingredient in seaweed. The average dietary intake of the Japanese is 8-10 mg of iodine per day. This amount easily clears the iodine intake necessary to saturate their thyroids. From an early age, including in utero, the fetus is well supplied with iodine. This likely is the reason the Japanese have the lowest incidence of congenital abnormalities and peri-natal problems in the world.

Japanese migrations

The Japanese have one of the lowest breast cancer, prostate cancer, and thyroid cancer rates in the world and only lately have had a small increase in the breast cancer rate thought to be related to the Westernization of their diet. But there have been a host of studies showing quite conclusively that the rate of breast cancer starts to go up markedly in the descendents of the first generation that migrates to North America. In the migrating generation there is little change in the incidence of breast cancer, but in each successive generation the breast cancer rate climbs rapidly to that of the host country such as the United States. In the light of mechanism suggested here, children of the first migrants would start to decrease their dietary intake of seaweed from that of their parents who did the migrating. The westernization of the children and the grand children would be complete within a couple of generations. So the iodine intake would then be the same as the North Americans and the breast cancer incidence becomes the same as the North Americans. The Japanese story is the most conspicuous, but similar stories happen to other migrating races.

Small thyroids in Iceland

If we continue with the thought that iodine deficiency makes thyroids enlarge to 20 grams or more, we should examine the meaning of a population with small thyroids. Japanese thyroid glands are about the smallest in the world in keeping with their high iodine intake. But what of a country that has thyroid glands smaller than even the Japanese? This happened in Iceland in the early part of the century up until about the WWI. The thyroid glands of the Icelandic people averaged 12 grams in the females and 14 grams in the males. This is the lowest weight of a thyroid gland recorded for any country in the world. It appears that this came about from the fishing industry, the main economic machine of Iceland. In the early part of the 1900s the leftover fish parts were ground up and given to the dairy cows as part of their feed. In turn the mammary glands of the dairy cows as is common for all mammals, concentrated the iodine from the left over fish into the milk. The milk of the Icelandic must have been high enough in iodine to saturate the thyroid gland. That means all of the young people, especially the young women, would have had high iodine intake at the time of breast development. As a consequence, the breast cancer rate was as low as or lower than the Japanese. A rate no other country has ever accomplished.

However, during the 40s and 50s the competition for the fishing rights off the shores of Iceland led to a much more efficient harvesting system with big ships and ever more carefully monitored distribution of the fish parts. By the 1960s, every part of the fish had a pre-designated country it was going to. Fish-meal, although still given to the cows, was given in measured amounts so as to follow the international standards of iodine intake. During this period the breast cancer rate rose by 10 times to that of the highest level in the United States. By lowering the iodine content of the milk to the accepted standards which are the same as those in the United States, a level which is known to only prevent goiters, the level of breast cancer went through a transition era of rapidly rising rates by ten times. Never in the world had such a huge drop in dietary iodine occurred on a national level, from very high levels to world-wide standardized levels. Only changes in iodine in descendants of migrating Japanese to North America compares with this.

One puzzling problem relates to lower incidence of breast cancer in southern climates. Countries with warmer climates did not appear to suffer the same breast cancer rate as northern countries like Canada, United States and Scandinavia with the exception of Japan and Iceland before WWII. But if we remember that the second phase of the cancer problem is related to tissue thyroid hormone then it becomes clearer. In the original description of severely hypothyroid patients, (myxedema) were described in the Committee report of 1888, there was no treatment for these people. The only treatment of any use to these very low thyroid patients was to move them to a warmer climate. All myxedematous patients did well if they moved to a warm climate. This means that the load on the thyroid system to maintain the body warmth is not needed. Therefore the amount of thyroid hormone freed up and made available for protecting the body from cancer invasion would be greater. In a sense, persons in warmer climates have a higher amount of thyroid available for tasks other than keeping warm. If so, then the breast cancer rate could be predictably lower in warmer climates and this is the case.

Haagersen was one of the last of this century's great American breast cancer surgeons who was trained in the manner of Halstead to do thorough total radical mastectomies. He was meticulous in keeping his records following his patients and chasing down the results of his own treatments. He and many others obtained excellent results using these methods. The massiveness of the surgery and the psychological damage to the patient eventually were part of the reasons this type of surgery was abandoned. During the years between 1915 and 1942 he worked at the Presbyterian Hospital in New York during which time he and his staff carefully took photographs, complete histories and made drawings to correlate with clinical signs of breast cancer and results of treatment and ultimate outcome of the patients. Together with Dr. Stout, the pathologist, they carefully analysed all the evidence to try to find the best treatment and understand the outcome of their treatments. In total 1544 breast cancer patients were followed in this manner completely through to the death of each patient. All data at the time was put into punch cards so it could be analysed. It turned out that four types of evidence were concerned with the clinical classification of the extent of the disease and the choice of treatment. They are:

1. The local extent of carcinoma in the breast and in the tissues covering it and situated beneath it on the chest wall.
2. The presence of and extent of metastases in the regional axillary, internal mammary, and supraclavicular lymph nodes.
3. The presence of distant metastases.
4. **Constitutional factors in the patient.**

The first three have been studied extensively ever since. The fourth factor was never mentioned again in Dr Haagersen's large book on breast cancer. Few have mentioned it in research reports. In fact, it has been largely ignored when our present treatments of radiation chemotherapy and surgery are potentially destabilizing to the constitution of the patient. If we think of the constitution in its true sense, then this is the make-up or functional habit of the body, determined by the genetic, biochemical and physiologic endowment of the individual, modified in great measure by environmental factors. Also, the constitution of a person means physical state as regards, vitality, health, strength, well being, etc

In 1971, Dr. R.I.S Bayliss, a famous endocrinologist was asked to speak at the Medical Society's Transactions. After many decades of treating thyroid conditions he was asked again how he could tell when a patient had adequate thyroid replacement. "I am often asked how the correct dose of thyroxine is determined. The answer is clinically by the patient's pulse rate, his sense of well-being, the texture of his skin, his tolerance of cold, his bowel function, and the speed with which his deep tendon reflexes relax." Is thyroid not the hormone capable of raising the constitution and well being of the patient? Any one can be brought up to the top of their constitutional capabilities when treated adequately with thyroid hormone. This would only be done by a clinical assessment, not blood tests, as there is no relation between the signs and symptoms of low thyroid disease, the TSH or the other related blood tests.

The treatment of thyroid cancer before the arrival of the TSH test was with sub-toxic doses. The dose of thyroid extract given rose until the patient had some symptoms of too much thyroid and then the dose lowered slightly below that. At these levels the body functions, including the immune system, are working at or near optimal rates for that individual. It goes without saying that these patients felt good and no side effects were reported.

The way to prevent breast cancer is with iodine. The way to turn around our breast cancer rates into a chronic disease is to use adjuvant thyroid hormone more freely to strengthen the patient's ability to deal with the disease both psychologically and physically. Surgical removal of the lesion still seems mandatory, the earlier the better. At the same time, a boost in overall constitutional factors with thyroid hormone will make the patient tolerate chemotherapy better and radiation much better than has been hitherto realized. Patients I have placed on normal doses of thyroid hormone prior to radiation have tolerated treatment better than most patients. This has also applied to chemotherapy. But the women who have not had these types of therapy have also done well.

The concepts put forward here are the result of prolonged observation and questioning of many patients. The general practitioner is in the best position of any profession in the world to observe the benefits and side effects of any treatment. The overall idea here is to try and approach breast cancer from a different viewpoint and from a different objective. It has long been thought to be important to rid every cancerous cell from the body. However, if we look at it differently so that we can just stop the cancer from growing, then it becomes nothing more than a process that can be stopped, which has only minor effects on the life of the individual.

In 1954, Dr. J. G. C. Spencer carried out a wide-ranging examination of the relation between thyroid and malignant disease. He concluded from all of his different findings that there was a strong relationship and he says it this way, "In coming to any conclusions regarding the possible association between malignant disease and thyroid function, it cannot be too strongly stressed that a low metabolic rate or insufficiency of thyroid substance can in no way be considered as a primary cause of cancer. Thyroid and related substances cannot therefore be considered as a cure for cancer. It is, however, suggested that thyroid function (or dysfunction) may be associated with a susceptibility or immunity to cancer. As such, thyroid might well be used as a therapeutic weapon, ancillary only to accepted surgical treatment."

"In the wider and perhaps more important field of preventive medicine, the possibility that an increased susceptibily to cancer occurs in those with a poor thyroid function leads for the first time to a real chance of adopting prophylactic measures against cancer on a wide scale. The measures adopted would be in the main those available against goitre in the young and adolescents, with the idea of building up healthy active thyroid glands during their period of development; and in adult life steps would be taken to maintain a good level of thyroid activity by ensuring that iodine is available in suitable quantities in food and drink, especially when middle life is reached and there is a natural tendency of the iodine level to fall. Only in such a way can an immunity be built up against the many carcinogenic substances which it is virtually impossible to avoid, largely due to the widespread use of coal and oil."

I believe Dr. Spencer had the right idea.

Figure 15

Biphasic nature of breast cancer

Progression from normal ducts

to invasive cancer

Fibrocystic disease

Cancer

    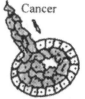

| Normal
Duct | Intraductal
Hyperplasia | Intraductal
hyperplasia
With Atypia | Intraductal
Carcinoma
in situ | Invasive
ductal
cancer |

Iodine in diet makes abnormalities
go back to normal

Thyroid
Hormone
Stops in
Connective
Tissue

Low iodine causes

Fibrocystic disease

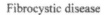
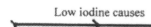

Breast Cancer References

1. Potten, C. S., Watson, R. J., Williams, G. T., Tickle, S., Roberts, S. A., Harris, M., & Howell, A. The effect of age and menstrual cycle upon proliferative activity of the normal human breast. Br J Cancer 58, 163-170. 1988.

2. Anderson, T. J., Ferguson, D. J., & Raab, G. M. Cell turnoverin the "resting" human breast: influence of parity, contraceptive pill, age and laterality. Br J Cancer 46, 376-382. 1982.

3. McCready, D. & Eskin, B. When the breasts are lumpy and painful. Patient Care Canada 7, 61-65. 1996.

4. Hutter, RV. Concensus meeting: Is fibrocystic disease of the breast precancerous? Arch Pathol Lab Med 110, 171-173. 1986.

5. Monson, R. R., Yen, S., & MacMahon, B. Chronic mastitis and carcinoma of the breast. Lancet July 31, 224-226. 1976.

6. Gullino, P. M. Natural history of breast cancer. Cancer 39, 2697-2703.

7. 1977.

8. Cullen, K. J., Allison, A., Martire, I., Ellis, M., & Singer, C. (1992). Insulin-Like Growth Factor Expression in Breast Cancer Epithelium and Stroma. Breast.Cancer Res.Treat., 22, 21-29.

9. Hutter, R. V. Goodbye to "Fibrocystic disease". The New England Journal of Medicine 312, 179-181. 1985.

10. Tobiassen, T., Rasmussen, T., Doberl, A., & Rannevik, G. Danazol treatment of severely symptomatic fibrocystic breast disease adn long term follow up — The Hjorring project. Acta Obstet Gynecol Scand Suppl 123, 159-176. 1984.

11. Fentiman, I. S. Prospects for the prevention of breast cancer. Ann Rev Med 43, 181-194. 1992.

12. Devitt, J. E. Abandoning fibrocystic disease of the breast: timely end of an era. Can.Med.Assoc.J. 134, 217-218. 1986.

13. Love, S. M., Gelman, R. S., & Silen, W. Fibrocystic "Disease" of the breast —a nondisease? The New England Journal of Medicine 307, 1010-1014. 1982.

14. Love, R. R. Approaches to the prevention of breast cancer. J Clin Endocr Metab 80, 1757-1760. 1995.

15. Benign and malignant proliferative epithelial lesions of the breast; a review. Eur J Cancer Clin Oncol 19, 1717-1720. 1985.

16. Davis, H. H., Simons, M., & Davis, J. B. Cystic Disease of the breast: relationship to carcinoma. Cancer 8, 957-978. 1964.

17. Dupont, W. D. & Page, D. L. Risk factors for breast cancer in women with proliferative breast disease. The New England Journal of Medicine 312, 146-151. 1985.

18. Ashikari, R., Huvos, A. G., Snyder, R. E., Lucas, J. C., Hutter, R. V., McDivitt, R. W., & Schottenfeld, D. A clinicopahtologic study of atypical lesions of the breast. Cancer 33, 310-317. 1974.

19. Kramer, W. M. & Rush, B. F. Mammary duct proliferation in the elderly. Cancer 31, 130-137. 1973.

20. Cook, M. G. & Rohan, T. E. (1985). The pathoepidemiology of benign proliferative epithelial disorders of the female breast. J Pathol, 146, 1-15.

21. Page, D. L. & Dupont, W. D. (1990). Anatomic markers of human premalignancy and risk of breast cancer. Cancer, 66, 1326.

22. Bodian, C. A., Perzin, K. H., Lattes, R., Hoffmann, P., & Abernathy, T. G. (1993). Prognostic significance of benign

proliferative breast disease [see comments]. Cancer, 1993 Jun 15;71, 3896-3907.

23. Webber, W. & Boyd, N. (1986). A critique of the methodology of studies of benign breast disease and breast cancer. J Natl Cancer Inst, 77, 397-404.

24. Townsend, C. M. (1980). Breast Lumps. Clinical symposia Ciba, 32, 3-32.

25. Wellings, S. R. Development of human breast cancer. Advan Cancer Res 31, 287-314. 1980.

26. Tulinius, H. & Sigvaldason, H. (1982). Trends in incidenceof female breast cancer in the Nordic countries. In K.Magnus (Ed.), Trends in Cancer Incidence (pp. 235-247). Washington: Hemisphere Publishing Corporations.

27. Hutchison, W. B., Thomas, D. B., & Hamlin, W. B. (1980). Risk of breast cancer in women with benign breast disease. J Natl Cancer Inst, 65, 13-20.

28. Wellings, S. R., Jensen, H. M., & Marcum, R. G. An atlas of subgross pathology of the human breast with special reference to possible precancerous lesions. J Nat.Cancer Inst. 55, 231-273. 1975.

29. Rosen, P. P., Braun, D. W., & Kinne, D. E. (1980). The clinical significance of pre-invasive breast carcinoma. Cancer, 46, 919-925.

30. Haagensen, D. E. (1991). Is cystic disease related to breast cancer? Am J Surg Pathol, 15, 687-694.

31. Dupont, W. D. & Page, D. L. (1985). Risk factors for breast cancer in women with proliferative breast disease. The New England Journal of Medicine, 312, 146.

32. Connolly, J. L. & Schnitt, S. J. (1993). Benign breast disease—resolved and unresolved issues. Cancer, 71, 1187-1189.

33. Rosen, P. P. (1991). "Borderline" breast lesions (letter). Am J Surg Pathol, 15, 1100-1102.

34. Moseson, M., Koenig, K. L., Shore, R. E., & Pasternack, B. S. (1993). The influence of medical conditions associated with hormones on the risk of breast cancer [published

erratum appears in Int J Epidemiol 1994 Dec;23(6):1330].
International Journal of Epidemiology, 22, 1000-1009.

35. Boynes, A. R., Cole, E. N., & Griffiths, K. Plasma prolactin in breast cancer. Eur J Cancer 9, 99-102. 1973.

36. Kodlin, D., Winger, E. E., Morgenstern, N. L., & et al (1977). Chronic mastopathy and breast cancer A follow up study. Cancer, 39, 2603-2607.

37. Lubin, F., Wax, Y., Ron, E., Black, M., Chetrit, A., Rosen, N., Alfandary, E., & Modan, B. (1989). Nutritional factors associated with benign breast disease etiology: a case-control study. American Journal of Clinical Nutrition, 50, 551-556.

38. Hellman, S. Dogma and inquisition in medicine. Cancer 71, 2430-2433. 1993.

39. Krieger, N. & Hiatt, R. A. (1992). Risk of breast cancer after benign breast diseases: variation by histologic type, degree of atypia, age of biopsy, and length of follow up. Am J Epidemiol., 135, 619-631.

40. Bodian, C. A. (1993). Benign breast disease, carcinoma in situ, and breast cancer risk. Epidemiol.Rev., 15, 177-187.

41. Goodwin, W. H., Miller, T. R., Sickles, E. A., & et al (1990). Lack of correlation of clinical breast examination with high risk histopathology. American Journal of Medicine, 89, 752-756.

42. Dupont, W. D., Parl, F. F., Hartmann, W. H., & et al (1993). Breast cancer risk associated with proliferative breast disease and atypical hyperplasia. Cancer, 71, 1258-1265.

43. Skrabanek, P. False premises and false promises of breast cancer screening. Lancet Aug 10, 316-320. 1985.

44. Gallager, H. S. & Martin, J. E. The study of mammary carcinoma by mammography and whole organ sectioning. Cancer 23, 855-873. 1969.

45. Black, M. M., Barclay, T. H., Cutler, S. J., Hankey, B. F., & Asire, A. J. Association of atypical characteristics of benign breast lesions with subsequent risk of breast cancer. Cancer 29, 338-343. 1972.

46. Eskin, B. A. (1970). Iodine metabolism and breast cancer. Trans NY Acad Sci, 32, 911-947.

47. Eskin, B. A., Grotkowski, C. E., Connolly, C. P., & Ghent, W. R. (1995). Different tissue responses for iodine and iodide in rat thyroid and mammary glands. Biol Trace Element Res, 49, 9-19.

48. Eskin, B. A., Grotkowski, C. E., Connolly, C. P., & Ghent, W. R. (1995). Different tissue responses for iodine and iodide in rat thyroid and mammary glands. Biological Trace Element Research, 49, 9-19.

49. Ghent, W. R., Eskin, B. A., Low, D. A., & Hill, L. P. (1993). Iodine replacement in fibrocystic disease of the breast. Can J Surg, 36, 453-460.

50. Eskin, B. A., Shuman, R., Krouse, T., & Merion, J. A. (1975). Rat mammary gland atypia produced by iodine blockade with prechlorate. Cancer Res, 35, 2332-2339.

51. Strum, J. M. (1978). Site of iodination in rat mammary gland. Anat Rec, 192, 235-244.

52. Strum, J. M., Phelps, P. C., & McAtee, M. M. (1983). Resting human female breast tissue produces iodinated proteins. J Ultrastruct Res, 84, 130-139.

53. Eskin, B. A., Sparks, C. E., & LaMont, B. I. The intracellular metabolism of iodine in carcinogeneis. Biol Trace Element Res 1, 101-117. 1979.

54. Krouse, T. B., Eskin, B. A., & Mobini, J. Arch Pathol Lab Med 103, 631-634. 1979.

55. Thorpe, S. M. (1976). Increased uptake of iodide by hormone-responsive compared to hormone-dependent mammary tumors in GR mice. Int J Cancer, 18, 345-350.

56. Aquino, T. I. & Eskin, B. A. (1972). Rat breast structure in altered iodine metabolism. Arch Pathol, 94, 280-285.

57. Eskin, B. A., Krouse, T. B., Modhera, P. R., & Mitchell, M. A. (1986). Etiology of mammary gland pathophysiology induced by iodine deficiency. In G.Medeiros-Neto & E. Gaitan (Eds.), Frontiers in thyroidology, Proceedings of the Ninth International Congress, (pp. 1027-1031). New York: Plenum.

58. Ciatto, S. & Bonardi, R. Is breast cancer ever cured? Follow-up study of 5623 cancer patients. Tumori 77, 465-467. 1991.

59. Devitt, J. E. Breast cancer: have we missed the forest because of the tree? Lancet 344, 734-735. 1994.

60. Lee, K., Bradley, R., Dwyer, J., Lee, S. L., & ' (1999). Too much or too little: The implication of current Iodine intake in the United States. Nutrition Reviews, 57, 177-181.

61. Fisher, E. R., Gregorio, R. M., & Fisher, B. (1975). The pathology of invasive breast cancer. A syllabus derived from findings of the National Surgical Breast Cancer Project (Protocol no. 4). Cancer, 36, 1-85.

62. Adami, H. O. & Killander, D. (1984). Prediction of survival in breast cancer. Principles and current status of hormone receptors and DNA content as prognostic factors. Acta Chirurgica Scandinavica - Supplementum, 519, 25-34.

63. Kelsey, J. L. & Berkowitz, G. S. Breast cancer epidemiology. Cancer Res 48, 5615-5623. 1988.

64. Madigan, M. P., Zeigler, R. G., Benichou, J., Byrne, C., & Hoover, R. N. Proportion of breast cancer cases in the United Startes explained by well-established risk factors. J Nat.Cancer Inst. 87, 1681-1685. 1995.

65. Kelsey, J. L. A review of teh epidemiology of human breast cancer. Epidemiol.Rev. 1, 74-108. 1979.

66. Buell, P. J. Changing incidence of breast cancer in Japanese-American women. J Natl Cancer Inst 51, 1479-1483. 1973.

67. Inoue, R., Fukutomi, T., Jshijima, T., Matsumoto, Y., Sugimura, T., & Nagao, M. Germline mutation of BRCA1 in Japanese breast cancer families. Cancer Res 55, 3521-3524. 1995.

68. Gallager, H. S. & Martin, J. E. Early phases in the development of breast cancer. Cancer 24, 1170-1178. 1969.

69. Qualheim, R. E. & Gall, E. A. Breast carcinoma with multiple sites of origin. Cancer 10, 460-468. 1957.

70. Hunter, D. J., Spiegelman, D., Adami, H. O., Beeson, L., van den Brant, P. A., Folsom, A. R., & Fraser, G. E. Cohort studies of fat intake and the risk of breast cancer a pooled

analysis. The New England Journal of Medicine 334, 356-361. 1996.

71. Miller, A. B., Kelly, A., Choi, N. W., Matthew, V., Morgan, R. W., Munan, L., Burch, J. D., Feather, J., Howe, G. R., & Jain, M. A study of diet and breast cancer. Amer J Epidemiology 107, 499-509. 1978.

72. Wiseman, R. A. (2000). Breast cancer hypothesis: a single cause for the majority of cases. J Epidemiol Community Health, 54, 851-858.

73. Weisburger, J. H., Reddy, B. S., Cohen, L. A., Hill, P., & Wynder, E. L. (1982). Mechanisms of promotion in nutritional carcinogenesis. Carcinogenesis, a Comprehensive Survey;1982;7, 175-182.

74. Garnick, M. B. & Fair, W. R. Combating prostate cancer. Scientific American [December], 74-83. 1998.

75. Riggs, J. E., Schochet, S. S. J., & Gutmann, L. (1984). Benign focal amyotrophy. Variant of chronic spinal muscular atrophy. Archives of Neurology, 41, 678-679.

76. Haggie, J. A. & et al. (1987). Fibroblasts from relatives of patients with heriditary breast cancer show fetal-like behavior in vitro. Lancet, i, 1455-57.

77. Adami, H. O., Rimsten, A., Stenkvist, B., & Vegelius, J. (1978). Reproductive history and risk of breast cancer: a case-control study in an unselected Swedish population. Cancer, 41, 747-757.

78. Adami, H. O., Hansen, J., Jung, B., & Rimsten, A. J. (1980). Age at first birth, parity and risk of breast cancer in a Swedish population. British Journal of Cancer, 42, 651-658.

79. MacMahon, B., Cole, P., Lin, T. M., Lowe, C. R., Mirra, A. P., Ravnihar, B., Salber, E. J., Valaoras, V. G., & Yuasa, S. Age at first birth and breast cancer risk. Bull Wld Hlth Org. 43, 209-221. 1970.

80. Ziegler, R. G., Hoover, R. N., Pike, M. C., Hildesheim, A., Nomura, A. M., West, D. W., Wu-Williams, A. H., Kolonel, L. N., & Horn-Ross, P. L. Migration patterns and breast cancer risk in Asian-American women. J Nat.Cancer Inst. 85, 1819-1827. 1993.

81. Katagari, T., Emi, M., Ito, I., Kobayashi, K., Yoshimoto, M., Iwase, T., Kasumi, F., Miki, Y., Skolnick, M. H., & Nakamura, Y. Mutations in the BRCA1 gene in Japanese breast cancer patients. Human Mutation 7, 334-339. 1996.

82. Mittra, I., Perrin, J., & Kumaoka, S. Thyroid and other autoantibodies in British and Japanese women: an epidemiological study of breast cancer. BMJ 1, 257-259. 1976.

83. Sigurjonsson, J. (1940). The small-size Iodine-Rich thyroid. In <u>Studies on the human thyroid gland in Iceland</u> (pp. 279-282). Reykjavik.

84. Carter, C. L., Corle, D. K., Micozzi, M. S., & e (1988). A propective study of the development of breast cancer in 16,692 women with benign breast disease. <u>Am J Epidemiology, 128,</u> 467-477.

85. Gray, G. E., Pike, M. C., Hirayama, T., Tellez, J., Gerkins, V., Brown, J. B., Casagrande, J. T., & Henderson, B. E. (1982). Diet and hormone profiles in teenage girls in four countries at different risk for breast cancer. <u>Preventive Medicine, 1982 Jan;11,</u> 108-113.

86. Steingrimsdottir, L. (1993). Nutrition in Iceland. <u>Scand Ju Nutri, 37,</u> 10-12.

87. Bjarnason, O., Day, N., Snaedal, G., & Tulinius, H. The effect of year of birth on the breast cancer age-incidence curve in Iceland. Int J Cancer 13, 689-696. 1974.

88. Randall, H. (1996). Iceland's bounty. <u>Canadian Wildlife,</u> 12-19.

89. Bjarnason, O., Day, N., Snaedal, G., & Tulinius, H. (1974). The effect of year of birth on the breast cancer age-incidence curve in Iceland. <u>International Journal of Cancer, 1974 May 15;13,</u> 689-696.

90. Crooks, J., Tulloch, M. I., Turnbull, A. C., Davidson, D., Skulason, T., & Snaedal, G. Comparative incidence of goitre in pregnancy in Iceland and Scotland. Lancet Sept 23, 625-627. 1967.

91. Alexander, W. D., Gudmundsun, T. V., Bluhm, M. M., & Harden, R. M. Studies of iodine metabolism in Iceland. Acta Endocr 46, 679-683. 1964.

92. Maunsell, E., Brisson, J., & Deschenes, L. Social support and survival among women with breast ca. Cancer 76, 631-637. 1995.

93. Townsend, C. M. (1988). Management of breast cancer. Ciba Foundation Colloquia on Endocrionology 3-32.

94. Love, S. M. & Lindsay, K. (1995). Dr. Susan Love's Breast Cancer book. (Second ed.) Cambridge, Massachusetts: Perseus Books.

95. Rawson, R. W. The thyroid gland. [18], 35-63. 1966. Ciba Serial (Book,Monograph)

96. Williams, R. H. & Bakke, J. L. (1962). The Thyroid. In R.H.Williams (Ed.), Textbook of Endocrinology (3 ed., pp. 96-281). Philadelphia: W.B. Saunders Company.

97. Beaston, G. T. On the treatment of inoperaable cases of carcinoma of the mamma: Suggestions for a new method of treatment, with illustrative cases. Lancet 2, 104-107-162-165. 1896.

98. Liechty, R. D., Hodges, R. E., & Burket, J. (1963). Cancer and thyroid function. JAMA, 183, 30-32.

99. Pories, W. J., Mansour, E. G., & Strain, W. H. (1972). Trace elements that act to inhibit neoplastic growth. Annals of the New York Academy of Sciences, 199, 265-273.

100. Shering, S. G., Zbar, A. P., Moriarty, M., McDermott, E. W., O'Higgins, N. J., & Smyth, P. P. (1996). Thyroid disorders and breast cancer. European Journal of Cancer Prevention, 5, 504-506.

101. Morabia, A., Szklo, M., Stewart, W., Schuman, L., Thomas, D. B., & Zacur, H. A. (1992). Thyroid hormones and duration of ovulatory activity in the etiology of breast cancer. Cancer Epidemiology, Biomarkers & Prevention, 1, 389-393.

102. Mittra, I. & Hayward, J. L. (1974). Hypothalamic-pituitary-thyroid axis in breast cancer. Lancet, 1, 885-888.

103. Martinez, L., Castilla, J. A., Gil, T., & et al (1995). Thyroid hormones in fibrocystic disease. Eur J Endocrinol, 132, 673-676.

104. Bulbrook, R. D., Thomas, B. S., Farah, J. M., Jr., & Hayward, J. L. (1981). A prospective study of the relation between thyroid function and subsequent breast cancer. In M.C.Pike, P. K. Siiteri, & C. W. Welsch (Eds.), Hormone and breast cancer Banbury report (pp. 131-140). Cold Spring Harbor: Cold Spring Harbor Laboratory.

105. Wynder, E. L., Bross, I. J., & Hirayama, T. (1960). A study of the epidemiology of cancer of the breast. Cancer, 13, 559-601.

106. Peter, F., Pickardt, C. R., & Breckwoldt, M. Thyroid hormones in benign breast disease. Cancer 56, 1982-1085. 1985.

107. Vorherr, H. Thyroid function in benign and malignant breast disease. Eur J Cancer Clin Oncol 22, 301-307. 1986.

108. Smyth, P. P. Thyroid disease and breast cancer. J Endocrin Invest 16, 396-401. 1993.

109. Thomas, B. S. & et al. (1983). Thyroid function in early breast cancer. Eur J Cancer Clin Oncol, 19(9), 1213-1219.

110. Estes, N. C. (1981). Mastodynia due to fibrocytic disease of the breast controlled with thyroid hormone. Am J Surg, 142(6), 764-766.

111. Moosa, A. R., Price-Evans, D. A., & Brewer, A. C. (1973). Thyroid status and breast cancer. Ann R Coll Surg Engl, 53, 178-188.

112. Edelstyn, G. A., Lyons, A. R., & Welbourn, R. B. (1958). Thyroid function in patients with mammary cancer. Lancet, 1(7022), 670-671.

113. Nasset, E. S. & et al. (1959). Inhibition of gastric secretion by thyroid preparations. Am J Physiol, 196, 1262-1265.

114. Backwinkle, K. & Jackson, A. S. (1964). Some features of breast cancer and thyroid deficiency. Cancer, 17, 1174.

115. Schottenfeld, D. (1968). The relationship of breast cancer to thyroid disease. J Chron Dis, 21, 303.

116. Stoll, B. A. (1965). Breast cancer and hypothyroidism. Cancer, 18, 1431-1436.

117. Thomas, B. S., Bulbrook, R. D., Russell, M. J., Hayward, J. L., & Millis, R. Thyroid function in early breast cancer. Eur J Cancer Clin Oncol 19, 1213-1219. 1983.

118. Stoll, B. A. (1962). A clinical trial of triiodothyronine as a hormone potentiator in advanced breast cancer. British Journal of Cancer, 16, 436-440.

119. Adamopoulos, D. A. & et al. (1986). Thyroid disease in patients with benign and malignant mastopathy. Cancer, 57(1), 125-128.

120. Humphrey, L. J. & et al. (1964). The relationship of breast cancer disease to thyroid disease. Cancer, 17, 1170-1173.

121. Chalstrey, L. J. & et al. (1966). High incidence of breast cancer in thyroid cancer patients. Brit J Cancer, 20, 670-675.

122. Lyons, A. R. & et al. (1965). Thyroid hormone as a prophylactic agent following radical treatment of breast cancer. Brit J Cancer, 19, 116-121.

123. Moossa, A. R. & et al. (1973). Thyroid status and breast cancer. Reappraisal of an old relationship. Ann R Coll Surg Engl, 53, 178-188.

124. Mittra, I., Hayward, J. L., & McNeilly, A. S. (1974). Hypothalamic-pituitary-thyroid axis in breast cancer. Lancet, 1, 889-891.

125. Emery, E. W. & Trotter, W. R. Triiodothyronine in advanced breast cancer. Lancet feb 16, 358-359. 1963.

126. Spencer,J.G.(1954) The influence of the thyroid in malignant disease. British J of Cancer7:8 393-411.

ISBN 155212884-9

Printed in the United States
By Bookmasters